TROUBLED WATER

Also by Seth M. Siegel

Let There Be Water: Israel's Solution for a Water-Starved World

TROUBLED WATER

WHAT'S WRONG WITH WHAT WE DRINK

SETH M. SIEGEL

THOMAS DUNNE
BOOKS

NEW YORK

First published in the United States by Thomas Dunne Books, an imprint of
St Martin's Publishing Group

TROUBLED WATER. Copyright © 2019 by Seth M. Siegel. All rights reserved.
Printed in the United States of America. For information, address St. Martin's
Press, 120 Broadway, New York, NY 10271.

www.thomasdunnebooks.com

The Library of Congress Cataloging-in-Publication Data is available upon request.

ISBN 978-1-250-13254-3 (hardcover)
ISBN 978-1-250-132550-(ebook)

Our books may be purchased in bulk for promotional, educational, or business
use. Please contact your local bookseller or the Macmillan Corporate and Premium Sales Department at 1-800-221-7945, extension 5442, or by email at
MacmillanSpecialMarkets@macmillan.com.

First Edition: October 2019

10 9 8 7 6 5 4 3 2 1

For Rachel,
and for our children,
with love beyond measure

Contents

CONTENTS

Preface

LATE IN THE research for what became *Let There Be Water*, my book about solutions for the coming global water scarcity, I stumbled upon what became the topic of this book. I was interviewing Professor Dror Avisar, a hydrochemist who heads Tel Aviv University's Water Research Center, and he raised a concern that, with a handful of exceptions, it was common to find contaminants in drinking water. With so many pharmaceutical products and industrial chemicals all around us, and with a lack of protective measures taken by most water utilities, the level of contamination was growing worse. He said that this wasn't a theory but a scientific fact, even if one not yet known by the public.

What Professor Avisar didn't know, he said, was what the long-term effect on human health would be from the exposure to so many contaminants in our drinking water. He lamented that more research wasn't being done to help figure out where danger might lie. The professor also said that much greater effort was needed in upgrading wastewater and drinking water treatment facilities. We had the engineering and scientific know-how to remove the contaminants that researchers had concluded were present. But we weren't using them because of a reluctance to spend what he guessed was a few dollars per person per month to solve the problem.

With my curiosity piqued, soon after I finished *Let There Be Water* I began reading about contaminants in drinking water. That led to my calling several national authorities to ask about academic papers they had written. If at first my investigation was limited to scientific elements, I was soon eager to also know how Congress has tried to legislatively handle the challenge, what the EPA was (or often, wasn't) doing, and how local drinking water utilities addressed the problem, among other areas.

After *Let There Be Water* came out, I began to get invitations to speak. My favorite part of what grew to be hundreds of talks was the Q&A session that followed my formal remarks. Although my book was about available water *quantity,* invariably someone in the audience wanted me to speak about drinking water *quality.* The consistency of the question led me to realize that concerns about drinking water safety were more widely felt than I imagined. I saw that many people had a sense that something was awry in America's drinking water. Between my own interest and what I saw as widespread public concern, before too long I had the subject for what evolved into *Troubled Water.*

What *Troubled Water* is not and does not aspire to be is an academic work targeted at a limited audience of professors and graduate students. Although I spent nearly two years reading academic papers and interviewing many professors and drinking water industry professionals to prepare for the writing of this book, the intended audience for it is intelligent readers who care about public affairs. Anyone who wants more is urged to dig into the endnotes and bibliography, to visit the book's website, or even to contact me. But no one need come to this book with prior knowledge about the subject or, indeed, any science background at all.

If *Troubled Water* is not an academic work, it is also not intended as an encyclopedic compendium of waterborne contaminants. That there are many other contaminants I could have chosen in the place of those identified and discussed here says less, I hope, about gaps in this book and more about the scope of the problem. The contaminants and challenges discussed here are each significant in their own right, but are also intended as an example of how our system has failed to keep up with growing insight on the public health effect of what is in our drinking water.

Even a casual look at this book will make clear that there is hardly a reference to the drinking water of other countries. There are three points about the editorial decision to be U.S.-centric in this book that I'd like to make. First, it was vexing enough to learn the legislative and regulatory framework for contaminants in my native country. Learning the same for several other countries would have delayed my efforts in getting this book out, something I was reluctant to do given the problems I believe need fixing in the U.S. Second, the water quality of countries outside of the U.S. has a serious impact on our health. It is from many of those countries that we get our fruit, vegetables, spices, fish, and other edibles. When we eat those foods, we are importing the drinking water health codes of those countries. And third, it would be an honor if authors in other countries wanted to use this book as a template for a book of their own about their country's drinking water. In some places, the drinking water is better than in the U.S. and, I suspect, in many places it is far worse. Everyone everywhere deserves the right to drink water without fear of contamination.

My ambitious goal for *Troubled Water* is to help launch a movement that will push for better water policies and safer drinking water than we now enjoy. Drinking water quality is an issue that gets far too little coverage by the media or discussion by elected officials and leaders of civil society. Without that attention, the changes needed will never occur. In that, I hope that every reader becomes an advocate for more effort and spending on drinking water issues. If so, it won't be long before every elected official concludes that drinking water is an important subject. Once that happens, we will have safer drinking water and a better system to deliver it. If *Troubled Water* helps to foster new laws, more health-focused regulations, significantly more research, and the adoption of needed technology in purifying drinking water, I will feel rewarded for my efforts.

I'd also like to have many partners in this effort. Please feel free to be in touch, and, most of all, to share your ideas. I look forward to hearing from you at www.TroubledWater.us.

New York City
May 2019

Introduction

EVEN WITH THE rise of bottled water as an alternative, most Americans still drink tap water. While there is generally no immediate mortal danger in doing so, the worry among respected scientists—several of whom the reader will meet in this book—is that contaminants often found in drinking water are disrupting the body's systems. Among other problems, some of these contaminants have been shown to cause cancer and cardiovascular disease, lead to hormonal disruptions linked to long-term health problems, harm children's brain development, and possibly trigger changes in our DNA that could later affect a child or grandchild.

Contaminants of one kind or another have been getting into our drinking water for many years. If previously much wasn't done about chemicals that would find their way into tap water, it could be explained away by saying that we just didn't know what was there. What is different now is that we have the scientific means to detect these toxic elements, and with other research tools, to come to a conclusion as to whether they are a threat to public health. Now, we know or can know, but there are significant impediments to doing what is needed to protect ourselves.

Drinking water in the U.S. is a victim not only of all of the many chemical compounds that find their way into drinking water as a contaminant, but also of an Environmental Protection Agency (EPA) that protects us inadequately. This book tells the story of how all of this came to pass, leaving us with drinking water that is less safe than we deserve. It also tells how, using known technology, and at an affordable price, we can have very clean and healthy water flowing in every pipe and from every sink.

The drinking water system we have today is the result of a failure of vision and a lack of technology, but also of institutions that—in their lethargy, in their adherence to the status quo, in their elevation of cost containment over public health, in their bias toward keeping chemicals in commerce as much as possible—have failed the public they are in place to serve.

There are, of course, smart, caring people across the government who touch water services and wish that they could do more—if only the system would let them. Likewise, there are some outstandingly managed state water programs and exemplary municipal water utilities. You will meet some of these people and water utilities in this book. But in a measure of how broken our system is, several people who deserved to be profiled—people at the EPA, in state government, and at local water utilities—were worried that their being named or even obliquely described in these pages would put them at risk of reprimand or of being fired because of their advocacy of new ideas. Apparently, offering even implied criticism of a broken system could be reason for retribution. Because of this, these individuals agreed to speak only in off-the-record interviews. If these people are the unidentified heroes of this book, happily there are others now out of government or in not-for-profit organizations willing to share their stories and ideas along with their names.

Although there are heroes in this book, it doesn't necessarily mean that there are villains. No one who is involved with the nation's drinking water is trying to deliver poor quality water. Everyone seems to want to do their best in what is a fractured and complex industry, where even a small mistake can lead to large numbers of people getting sick.

But if this book has no villains, perhaps it is fair to say that there are many culprits and bystanders. These people include some elected officials, some heads of regulatory agencies, and some of those running water utilities. On their watch, they have negligently or recklessly allowed America's drinking water to put our health at risk, even while new technologies and smart governance could have been improving it.

A few examples, much more of which you will soon read: The EPA isn't researching new contaminants often enough or quickly enough to stay ahead of the many chemicals in commerce and in our water. To the question, "What's in our water and with what effect on our health?," most of the time the answer is, "We don't know." Further, the EPA and state governments don't challenge the water utilities under their control and in their jurisdictions to spend more and to modernize their facilities and infrastructure. And the vast majority of water utilities have elevated keeping expenses down over making public health their top priority.

While the EPA's go-slow approach to the search for drinking water contaminants and its failure to effectively enforce current rules are the most significant causes of why America's drinking water is in decline, the scope of that inaction is similarly confounding. With more than 120,000 chemical compounds, pharmaceutical products, and plastics now in commerce, the EPA has only designated about ninety of them as problematic enough to be called "regulated." This is a status that triggers a requirement by the nation's water utilities to test for the presence of that contaminant and to then remove enough of it so that the water can be consumed without there being a health threat.

As startling as is the failure to not find even one hundred contaminants dangerous enough to be regulated in the nearly fifty years since the EPA was given authority to do so, that isn't the most shocking example of the EPA's lax oversight discussed in this book. The yet more amazing fact is this: Despite thousands of new potential water contaminants coming to market every year—and joining those other 120,000 chemical compounds, pharmaceutical products, and plastics—the last time the EPA regulated *any* new item as a drinking water contaminant was more than twenty years ago.

While, of course, the EPA shouldn't regulate a contaminant just to provide the appearance of activity, the opposite is also true: Contaminants shouldn't fail to be regulated just because the EPA hasn't developed a sense of urgency. The lack of timely research, on the one hand, and the inability to reach conclusions even after multiple rounds of research, on the other, is a symptom of misdirected legislation and poor execution by the EPA. There are at least dozens—and possibly hundreds—of contaminants that are known or suspected of being hazardous, but which have not been regulated. How this could be possible will soon be clear to the reader.

In addition to a limited amount of timely action by the EPA, drinking water suffers from a bloated number of water utilities. You could win a bet asking someone to guess how many water utilities there are in the U.S., because it defies logic and almost anyone's concept of efficiency. The impossibly large number—discussed in the book—is an impediment to the adoption of important technologies, replacing broken and failing pipes, retention of experienced engineers, and most important of all, delivery of the safest water possible.

Instead of relying on tap water, many Americans have turned to bottled water, now the most popular beverage in the U.S. While there may be some clever marketing by the soft drink companies at work, bottled water's success is due mostly to the failure of government and the water utilities to provide tap water that the public can trust. As discussed later in this book, over 90 percent of those who drink bottled water cite "safety" or "quality" as a reason for doing so. Proving this point, most bottled water is consumed within a few feet of a sink, and 60 percent of all bottled water sold is for use in people's homes. Driven by skepticism about the safety of their tap water, millions of Americans have defaulted to what has become an alternative drinking water system.

Whether bottled water is actually safer or healthier—it often isn't— is beside the point. If Americans are drinking bottled water when tap water is available, it is because they believe that the store-bought variety assures quality and safety—or even taste—that they can't get when they open their faucets. In what is an important message for our public officials, it also shows that people who have the means to do so are willing to pay more for their water, if they *believe* it will be of higher quality and safer to drink than the alternative.

In past generations, America laid more than 1.1 million miles of water mains to bring water from a central distribution point, branching out in every town and city in the country, to homes along the path. Our great-grandparents' generation figured out how to end waterborne epidemics that killed large numbers in short amounts of time. And our parents' and grandparents' generations built and paid for drinking water and wastewater treatment facilities all over the country, which, even if they are inadequate to address the drinking water challenges of today, met the needs, and were based on the scientific knowledge, of their time. In all of this, we have been great beneficiaries. Now, we have an opportunity to protect our health and the well-being of our children and grand-children by ensuring the cleanest water that technology allows.

We are at an inflection point similar to the years before the birth of America's environmental movement. People had a sense that something was amiss, but weren't organized and didn't know what to do to fix a natural world that seemed out of control—and a threat to their health. From out of that ferment came important environmental legislation, including federal drinking water laws. Similarly today, as confirmed by recent polls, Americans have a feeling that their drinking water isn't as good or safe as it should be. Just as with the rise of environmentalism, when the public comes together to demand healthy, safe drinking water, elected officials will respond.

Following is what we need to know so we can start demanding the water we can have, and deserve.

PART I

A BROKEN SYSTEM

One

WELCOME TO HOOSICK FALLS!

"Maybe it's something in the water."
—Michael Hickey

IT ISN'T CLEAR if John Hickey would have died of kidney cancer had he lived and worked somewhere other than Hoosick Falls. Like most of us, he thought the water in his town in upstate New York—located a short drive from the Vermont border—was clean and safe, or at least clean and safe enough. After he became sick and had a kidney removed in September 2010, and after his cancer came back a year or so later, killing him in February 2013, he still never had reason to doubt or wonder about the water in his town.

Even without visiting John Hickey's Hoosick Falls birthplace, you could accurately imagine it as a place with the iconic aura of small-town America, a place where the residents are friendly, courteous, and engaged in their community. A search for waterfalls there would prove futile—in the 1940s, the state government blew up the falls that had given the town half of its name as part of a flood prevention program—but otherwise the town (strictly speaking, a village) would likely conform to a visitor's idealized expectations.

That visitor could expect to find streets lined with attended-to front yards. The presence of a centrally located, well-manicured Little League baseball diamond with names of sponsoring local businesses painted on the outfield wall would, likewise, offer no surprise in this time-frozen Norman Rockwell tableau.

Outsiders who come from places where hyper-partisan politics are the norm might be shocked at first to learn that mayoral and village board elections in Hoosick Falls are always uncontested, but that, too, would soon make sense. As with thousands of other small towns and villages across America where community leaders have careers outside of politics and serve part-time in their elected positions, consensus is valued over party ideology and those in office believe they need to get along for the benefit of the public they are elected to serve. There's a reason why the make-believe town of Bedford Falls in the 1946 Jimmy Stewart–Frank Capra classic *It's a Wonderful Life* felt so familiar to movie audiences then and now: It evoked thousands of communities just like Hoosick Falls, all across the country.

Unfortunately, there was no guardian angel like the film's Clarence to save most of the real-world versions of Bedford Falls. By the 1950s, the glory days of small-town factories all across America began a steady decline. Companies started consolidating factory locations and adopting technologies that would reduce the need for workers. And in the decades that followed, U.S. manufacturers increasingly looked to Asia and lower-wage countries where, in a globalizing world, products could be made more cheaply. Many factories in that bucolic small-town America closed their doors, leaving generations of workers to fend for themselves in a new global economy.

But Hoosick Falls was luckier than others, at least at first. Just as other industries were shutting down in Hoosick Falls, the demand for Teflon, in its many forms, grew rapidly throughout the U.S. and around the world. A salesman from just over the Hoosick Falls border in Vermont looking to change careers correctly saw the synthetic material as his road to fortune. With factories already built but now empty, the salesman-turned-entrepreneur located his new Teflon manufacturing business in his adopted town.[1] One factory led to another, until the town hosted eleven facilities that made Teflon or integrated it into some other product.[2] Available buildings aside, Hoosick Falls also offered reliable factory hands like John Hickey who could work, at round-the-clock shifts, creating Teflon-coated sheeting for tents, elastic tape that could be used as a sealant, and other Teflon-covered or infused "miracle solutions."

A fourth-generation resident of his town, John Hickey was a model of industriousness and reliability. He grew up poor and in economically unstable circumstances, and he didn't want that for his wife and three children. Believing it was his responsibility to care for his community and family, he pushed himself at what most people would think was an uncompromising pace. By day, he drove a yellow school bus in Hoosick Falls. After some family time and early dinner, he'd grab a few hours of sleep and then, shaking off fatigue, would rush to his factory job on the 11 p.m. to 7 a.m. shift where—for thirty-two years—night after night he worked at a variety of jobs. On weekends, John drove for a limousine service just over the New York state line in Vermont.[3]

John came to be one of the most popular people in Hoosick Falls. Of Irish heritage, he had pale skin that burned easily, but, except when playing a round of golf on the local public course, he wasn't outside for long stretches. His face, and five-foot-ten-inch frame, which became stocky with the years, was a familiar sight to his fellow townspeople. Throughout Hoosick Falls, he was known for his kindness and easy laugh. Every morning before he'd begin his bus route, he would stop at Stewart's, the local convenience store, for coffee. It was his custom to pay for himself— and whoever was lucky enough to be standing on line immediately behind him. Each year at holiday season, John went shopping for toys and gifts for the children on his bus from poor families. "No one should be without a gift at Christmas," he would say when asked why he did it, but some who knew him said it was a reflection of the pain he felt from some meager Christmas mornings from his economically deprived childhood. John's sweet disposition and small acts of kindness clearly registered with his neighbors. When he died, more than one thousand people lined up on a freezing February afternoon, standing long out the door of the funeral home where John's wake was held.

Despite the grueling work schedule, his son, Michael, remembers his father rarely missed his own kids' school sporting events. Forgoing a chance to rest, John would arrange to drive the after-school bus for any Hoosick Falls Central School teams on which his children competed. John even found time to serve in one of the elective positions on the Hoosick Falls village board.

Among the village board's functions was overseeing the work of the town's drinking water department and its two employees. Without any-one being aware of it—not those two water workers, not the village board, not the local media, not the New York State government, not the U.S. government's Environmental Protection Agency, and surely not the village's residents—year after year, the Hoosick Falls aquifer from which the town drew its drinking water became ever more contaminated.

"Better Living Through Chemistry"

If you've ever used a Post-it note or Scotch tape, you've been a customer of the 3M Company. Just as likely, probably without realizing it, you've also been an indirect consumer of 3M's industrial products. Their prod-ucts are essential elements of so many manufactured items that, inten-tionally or not, nearly every person living in the modern world owns or uses products that were made using 3M chemicals and supplies.

Called Minnesota Mining and Manufacturing Company from its founding in 1902 until a branding makeover and name change in the com-pany's centennial year, 3M's foray into producing those ever-present yellow "stickies" and its all-purpose tape were accidental, even if hugely successful, departures from the company's origins. That business, as its descriptive, founding name implied, was dedicated to coming up with products for industrial users.

From nearly its first days—and long before this was common among corporations—3M placed an emphasis on research, encouraging staff to anticipate customer needs as well as spending heavily on traditional white lab coat scientific experimentation to develop new products. Never content with just selling commodity products to its customers, 3M had (and still has) a pipeline full of products and ideas, including in areas as diverse as health care, automotive manufacturing, textiles, and industrial products, among many others.[4]

Not every 3M product concept was fully developed in-house. In 1946, the company became interested in the work of Joseph Simons, then a chemistry professor at Penn State University. Simons had spent the World War II years working on secret projects involving military applications for fluorine, a naturally occurring chemical that was used in the production of nuclear weapons. Freed from the constraints of wartime secrecy, Simons began experimenting with and writing about a new idea in which the bonding of fluorine and carbon molecules might result in a super compound of uncommon strength and durability.[5]

In acquiring Simons's patents, no one at 3M initially knew what products would flow from his idea or who the customers for it might be, but their intuition was that they were onto something big. As such, 3M's management decided to put lots of resources into seeing where this could lead. After a few years and, at one point, the combined effort of more than one hundred researchers, 3M came up with a chemical with many uses that seemed to justify the enormous investment in money and laboratory personnel. From Simons's single-fluorine-based idea, many different chemical compounds were created. In one of its formulations, the newly developed product was one with a multisyllabic name— perfluorooctanoic acid—abbreviated as PFOA.[6]

PFOA seemed to be a wondrous formulation. Plastic, metal, or cloth treated with PFOA would become impervious to water, grease, or fatty substances, and also to any solvent that touched it. As remarkable, PFOA exceeded durability thresholds of other protective materials, demonstrating it could withstand very high temperatures without degrading. In one test after another, the compound proved to be long lasting to the point of being nearly indestructible. The bet taken on the professor's idea proved to be a brilliant one, with the opportunity for unimaginably huge financial returns.

Of course, 3M wasn't the only company that had research facilities with well-funded chemistry labs hosting scientists in pursuit of new products for industry and consumers. Started in 1802, exactly one hundred years before 3M opened its doors, DuPont was founded by a French-American chemist who figured out a sophisticated method for producing gunpowder. As America grew, DuPont grew with it. By the time the Civil War broke out, DuPont had such a preferred relationship with the U.S. military that half of the gunpowder purchased by the Union armies in the war came from DuPont factories.

DuPont wasn't just a military contractor, even if a large part of its early revenues came from sales of ingredients to make muskets, rifles, and cannons effective and lethal. It was a chemistry company that employed science in creating products for both America and the world. Regardless of how those products were used, DuPont positioned itself as a vehicle for science—and specifically chemistry—to make lives better and more enjoyable. Whether simply a marketing tool or a reflection of the company's mission or both, for nearly fifty years beginning in the mid-1930s, DuPont used the advertising slogan "Better Things for Better Living . . . Through Chemistry."[7]

As often happens in research laboratories, some inventions happen by chance. One such fortunate mishap occurred a few years after the adoption of the "Better Living Through Chemistry" catchphrase when, in 1938, a DuPont chemist accidentally invented a slippery, low-friction material that could withstand high heat. Similar to the 3M experience with PFOA, DuPont's scientists and product developers began to search for how this unusual compound—called polytetrafluoroethylene, or PTFE, for short—could be commercialized.[8]

After several years of on-again, off-again experimentation, DuPont found that it could apply a coating of PTFE to pots and pans with an interesting result. Once treated with PTFE, baked or fried food that would ordinarily stick to the cookware could be easily cleaned with a wet cloth and a bit of soap. In what was seen as a potential revolution in tedious kitchen chores, burnt or encrusted matter would slip off the skillet with minimal effort.

PTFE was what came to be known as Teflon. If it could be brought to market, it would have obvious appeal to homemakers or kitchen staff. But the Teflon of 1945 wasn't ready for commercial use. While DuPont could adhere a layer of PTFE on a frypan and make cleanup easy, the coating would become lumpy. Much more work would be required before DuPont could see a financial return on this investment.

A year of trial and error ensued, with the solution coming from 3M. By adding PFOA into the production of Teflon, the thin PTFE layer would remain even and smooth on the cookware. Although Teflon was a DuPont product, the essential element to make it marketable was supplied by 3M to their mutual benefit. In the late 1940s, DuPont introduced Teflon cookware and other treated products. DuPont's success was 3M's success.[9]

But 3M's success with PFOA didn't stop there. Thousands of products beyond Teflon cookware were created in the years that followed.

Heat-resistant wires and cables could be produced by adding PFOA to the plastic insulation, making them safer to use in many settings where containing heat is important, or even essential, like inside airplanes and spacecraft. High-performance ski wax was created by mixing paraffin and PFOA. Pizza boxes and microwaveable popcorn bags coated with PFOA were brought to market to prevent grease from saturating the cardboard and paper, resulting in less mess for the consumer. Specialty Teflon tape in an array of sizes was created for the plumbing industry to utilize in sealing pipe threads. Boots, outdoor apparel, backpacks, and tents—like those made with Gore-Tex fabrics treated with PFOA—kept the shoes, clothing, and camping equipment water repellent and stain resistant.[10] W. L. Gore, the company that owned the Gore-Tex brand, even developed dental floss embedded with these slippery compounds after workers trimming the PFOA-treated fabrics realized that strands of it were uncommonly effective in gliding between teeth.[11] And on and on.

As broad as was the universe of products embedded with PFOA, 3M scientists discovered that Professor Simons's fluorine building blocks could also be used to create other compounds like PFOS, a chemical cousin of PFOA, which became used as a firefighting agent at all U.S. military bases, and at fire departments around the world. In other forms, PFOS was found to create stain resistance, and carpets and textiles were treated with it. As with PFOA, PFOS was durable to the point of near indestructibility.

Consumers responded to the seemingly limitless uses for PFOA (including in Teflon) in new products. DuPont's "Better Living Through Chemistry" boast sounded on target. And with this consumer response, billions of dollars of new revenue were generated, helping to drive profits at 3M, DuPont, W. L. Gore, and many other companies.[12] It was a benefit for consumers, and a bonanza for these companies. It was also an opportunity for some small towns to revive their faltering manufacturing industries.

Teflon Comes to Hoosick Falls

With Teflon products becoming the backbone of the manufacturing base in Hoosick Falls, the PFOA embedded in it wasn't limited to the products made in the town. Over time, and through several pathways, PFOA made its way into Hoosick Falls's wells and drinking water.

Some of the Teflon factories—including one 400 yards up a slope from the town's main source of water—incinerated their waste, sending the nearly indestructible PFOA particles airborne.[13] The cinders would settle in the town's many open spaces—those pretty lawns and the manicured Little League field included—and when rain fell, the chemical would be drawn into the soil and groundwater, the latter of which was the source of Hoosick Falls's drinking water. The contamination of that groundwater—with no required testing for or filtration of PFOA before the water was distributed—would expose John Hickey and his family, and every town resident, to potential harm.

Propelled by gravity, groundwater—which is found in the tiny air pockets between grains of sand or soil—bends around clay and other impermeable objects. It keeps in motion until it gets trapped in some geological formation that doesn't let it move farther or until it is pumped out to be used for drinking or some other purpose. Invisible to us, groundwater can travel great distances, picking up contaminants along its journey. Once contaminated, the noxious groundwater can befoul previously pristine places.[14]

Sometimes, pollutants that are drawn into groundwater get degraded during the underground route because of heat or cold or the passage of time. In other instances, toxic substances in polluted groundwater get rendered harmless after contact with naturally occurring elements in the soil that neutralize the contaminant in a chemical reaction. But not PFOA. Just as the chemical survives incineration, PFOA also survives the encounter with a range of temperatures and soil conditions.[15] This may be why PFOA from Hoosick Falls's groundwater was found in private drinking water wells as far as ten miles outside of the town.[16]

Ironically, well-intentioned environmental regulations issued in the early 1980s made the Hoosick Falls groundwater contamination worse. In an attempt to improve air quality, every factory with an incinerator was obliged to install scrubbers in its smokestack. Once a week, maintenance workers at those Hoosick Falls factories—including the factory just up a slope from the town's aquifer—would remove the scrubbers, bring them outside, and hose them down. The filtered PFOA residue would be absorbed into the soil and the groundwater.

Even the town landfill became an entry point for contamination. The solid waste facility was used to bury some of the industrial trash from the town's factories, much of it containing PFOA. Over time, the waste would break down, but not the enduring chemical. Few landfills are completely watertight, and the one in Hoosick Falls was not. PFOA in the Hoosick Falls landfill leached into the soil and percolated into the groundwater.

While the factories were the primary cause of contamination, the groundwater flowing into the town's aquifer and nearby wells from several directions was its means of delivery. Incrementally and slowly, the groundwater grew more contaminated. As the groundwater provided the water for the town's wells, soon and likely for a long time before it was discovered, the wells fed a toxic brew into the faucets of every home in the village.

Despite the groundwater contamination, if you lived in Hoosick Falls, you had benefited economically from the Teflon factories going back to the mid-1950s. But the benefit came—even if invisibly—at a price. Those in Hoosick Falls were unwittingly and regularly ingesting PFOA, a chemical resistant to breaking down and being flushed out of the body once consumed. Had they known the full story, it is likely few in the pretty village would have been willing to pay the price.

Cause and Effect

Scarcely one hundred years ago, if someone drank tainted water—even in the world's largest and most modern cities—he or she could be dead a few days later from cholera or dysentery or other waterborne pathogens.[17] Unlike the disparity between rich and poor communities and nations today, these bacterial diseases made no distinction for wealth or class, striking down even the most famous and most affluent along with the poorest of the anonymous poor.[18] After millions had already died, scientists came to understand that death from cholera and dysentery could be brought to an end if a few simple techniques were used to treat water before drinking it.

Around the turn of the twentieth century, scientists came up with two solutions. First, before drinking it, a city's water would be filtered through sand to get rid of bacteria and viruses. A few years later, minuscule quantities of chlorine began being added to the drinking water, eliminating the pathogens in it before the microorganisms could kill their human hosts.

Once the bacteria that caused cholera and dysentery were discovered, and then these physical and chemical systems were developed to neutralize them, the chance of a quick death from drinking water was reduced to near zero. But sand filters and chlorine (and more recently, if still not found as broadly as it should, ultraviolet light) can provide a false sense of confidence. As effective as these treatments are at stopping cholera and most—but not all—other waterborne pathogen-driven diseases, they leave untouched the chemicals that are now found in drinking water.[19]

Unlike death by cholera, in which rapidly multiplying bacteria overwhelm the victim's body, it is impossible to definitively say that a given person has died from drinking water with PFOA or small amounts of some other industrial chemicals now found in drinking water. Although not waterborne, cigarettes offer a good analogy in helping to understand the threat from these contaminants, as well as the difficulty with establishing cause and effect, or, in scientific lingo, causality.

Few products have been as subjected to medical studies as has tobacco. Yet, after billions spent on research by industry and government, not even one smoker's lung cancer death can be specifically tied to cigarettes. What scientists can do is draw an inference, and say that smokers as a group are more likely to get lung cancer and to die from it than a similar group of nonsmokers. But even so, in that group of smokers, some will live past the age of life expectancy with never so much as a cough, and some in the group of nonsmokers will get lung cancer and die without ever having had a cigarette. No one's first puff necessarily dooms them that day, and daily smoking won't necessarily kill you, even after a long period of exposure. Even so, there is no doubt that smoking is unsafe generally, even if not universally. Accordingly, if we learn of a heavy smoker who has died of lung cancer, most would assume the smoker's behavior led to the disease—with or without definitive causality in his or her particular case.

In the same way, most chemical contaminants in our drinking water have a long latency period. Patterns can be detected, but there is still less certainty as to cause and effect than with, say, cholera or dying from swallowing a large dose of cyanide or by a pedestrian being hit by a speeding car. Because of the less easily observable cause and effect created by the long gap between exposure to a contaminant and getting sick, it leads scientists to wonder whether a particular waterborne contaminant, or perhaps a mix of them, caused, for example, a hormonal disorder in a teenager or a certain cancer in an adult. Even when scientists have well-informed hunches that a contaminant in drinking water is the cause, it is often impossible to know with certainty, at least with the scientific information—and research budgets—we now have at hand.[20] It would be easier, to be sure, if a straight line of cause and effect could be drawn from each of the contaminants to a defined health outcome akin to being able to say that Person A was exposed to Chemical B and shortly thereafter came down with Disease C.

Most of the time, though, connecting the link from Chemical B to Disease C can still be shown, even if indirectly. This is done primarily with two kinds of investigation. The first is population, or epidemiological. These tests utilize sophisticated statistical analysis that show trends isolating a specific contaminant and an undesirable outcome. The other is toxicological studies. These use animals as stand-ins for humans with the expectation that exposure to certain toxic elements will reveal the likelihood of a human becoming sick in the same way as the animal test subject.

As was definitively concluded about smoking, regardless of any potential ambiguity created by the lack of an absolute finding of cause and effect, the better course for general public health would be to remove all potentially harmful contaminants until scientific research proves them to be harmless. Some of the drinking water contaminants may prove to be benign, but the safer route is to have a higher level of caution, and to suspect some of these widely found contaminants as being as injurious to public health as cholera and other pathogens once found in drinking water, if only acting much more slowly.

Unlike what grew into a mass campaign to protect society from the effects of smoking, outside of a handful of not-for-profit organizations, charitable foundations, and municipal water systems, there are few advocates today for an all-out effort to assure that water is free of contaminants. Given that there is no substance so universally consumed, it is puzzling why these safe-water campaigners aren't widely joined by others concerned about the environment, health, consumer affairs, and other areas of civic engagement.

Equally puzzling is how a society so smitten with new products and technologies allows its drinking water treatment to be managed as if time froze soon after chlorine's use became standard. With nearly all of us drinking water that is purified using techniques that were established as much as a century ago—and long before so many laboratory-created synthetic chemicals began getting into our drinking water—we are like generals fighting the last war.

Certainly, it is still essential to kill off the pathogens that spread cholera and dysentery via our drinking water, but the weapons deployed in today's fight, the metaphorical bayonets and fixed artillery pieces, have scarcely changed from the Victorian age. What other major area of life—health care, transportation, energy production, or, for that matter, warfare—has remained essentially static in addressing over-the-horizon challenges?

To the extent government entities are addressing it at all, the effort to analyze and prevent potential long-term harm from waterborne chemical contamination is being done in a disjointed, underfunded way with confusion about priorities at all levels of government. This confused and badly coordinated system explains how John Hickey could have spent most of his adult life drinking tap water contaminated with PFOA, even when the danger of it was known by those who knew enough to ask.

"Maybe It's Something in the Water"

A year after John Hickey's death, his son, Michael Hickey, was still tormented by his father's gruesome final days. He blamed himself for his father's suffering because—possible harsh side effects notwithstanding—he had urged him to choose the most aggressive treatment option the specialists in Boston had offered. The proposed therapy failed. And in John's final days, he suffered more than he would have had he not challenged the terminal diagnosis with the aggressive treatment and instead opted for the pain-managed end offered to him as an alternative.

But it wasn't just his father's death and his agonizing final days that unsettled Michael. Something seemed amiss, starting with John's kidney cancer diagnosis. There was no family history of this kind of cancer, which, like many other cancers, often has a genetic link. Also troubling was that his father died nearly twenty years younger than both of his parents, Michael's grandparents. His father's cancer had been first found in 2009 when he was in his sixties, while both of John's parents lived into their late eighties. Since parental longevity is indicative of a child's life expectancy, there was no reason, Michael thought, for such a large gap between the age of death of his father and that of his father's parents. And then there was the matter of lifestyle. John never smoked or drank, even during his brief stint in the navy, and he was active with work and sports until his initial diagnosis and beyond. Yet, despite all of this and despite advances in medical care and treatment from his parents' generation to his, John got sick at sixty-six and was dead at seventy. Not young, but not, Michael thought, the full—or rightful—measure of his days.

There was something else that didn't add up. John Hickey wasn't the only one in Hoosick Falls to get sick with a terrible disease. People younger than his father were being diagnosed with cancers, thyroid diseases, and other serious infirmities where, as with his father, there had been no family history to suppose a predisposition to those illnesses. Even if no one was formally tracking all of these medical diagnoses and collecting data to attempt to detect a pattern, the small size of Hoosick Falls and the intimate sense of community made for rapid sharing of information. Adding to the gloomy feeling, some well-cared-for family dogs in town developed unexplained tumors and had to be put down while still in what would normally be their good years. Even if they had no data to prove it, the volume of bad news certainly gave the residents of Hoosick Falls the feeling that they were having an uncommonly unlucky run.

One evening in late February 2014, almost exactly a year after John Hickey's death, Michael received a phone call from a high school friend, Courtney Hamilton, who, like Michael, still lived in Hoosick Falls. She had more bad news to report: Isabel McGuire, a math teacher in the high school and a resident in the village, had just died of melanoma. She was forty-eight.

"Michael," she asked, more as an expression of alarm than expecting her question to lead to an answer, "what is going on here?"

At a loss for words and drawing on a familiar phrase, Michael said, "Maybe it's something in the water."

Michael can't remember if Courtney laughed, but his reply was meant as much to break the tension as to actually be responsive. Sitting in front of his computer as Courtney continued to speak, in a flash, Michael thought about the dominant industry in his town. He cradled the receiver between his shoulder and ear as he opened Google on his screen. He typed in the words "Cancer and Teflon." He blinked hard as links to reports and articles popped up. He scrolled his mouse over one of the entries listed, and clicked it open. The first thing in the report to catch his eye were the words: Kidney cancer.

Exercising remarkable restraint, Michael didn't share what he had just seen, having the presence of mind to want to know more before saying anything. He quickly got off the phone with Courtney, and began reading.

At Cazenovia College, the small, liberal arts school in New York's

Finger Lakes region a few hours' drive from Hoosick Falls that Michael had attended, he had been a business major, staying away from science courses. In the fifteen years since he had graduated, he had worked in one business-related job after another, currently making the daily forty-five-minute commute to Albany, New York's capital, where he was an insurance underwriter. Despite the lack of a science background, Michael used his evenings after the call with Courtney searching for and reading everything he could find on the effect of PFOA on human health. He read scientific studies, government reports, newspaper articles, and academic monographs. Before long, he knew enough to be concerned.

Nearly all of Michael's reading made mention of Parkersburg, West Virginia, a community that—like Hoosick Falls—had suffered unexplained diseases and other medical abnormalities in people and animals. And like Hoosick Falls, a DuPont factory where PFOA was used had long been a local employer. But unlike Hoosick Falls, a relentless lawyer sued DuPont in 1999 on behalf of some of the residents of Parkersburg, successfully demonstrating that the company had released PFOA into the nearby Ohio River and elsewhere, polluting the area's water resources from the 1950s until the early 2000s when the successful lawsuit forced DuPont to stop.[21]

As part of the settlement, DuPont paid a fine and was required to fund the creation of an impartial scientific panel to study the health effects of long-term exposure to PFOA. Remarkably, while this study was going on for eight years beginning in 2005, no one—not DuPont or the chemical industry trade association, nor the EPA or the New York State government—thought to alert other communities that had long been exposed to PFOA that, maybe, they should have their water tested. In 2014, and more than nine years after the West Virginia settlement, the residents of Hoosick Falls were still drinking water that, at best, had some questionable effects and, at worst, was the catalyst for personal, family, and communal tragedies.[22]

Michael Hickey's Education

Given Michael Hickey's lack of science education, his first instinct was to seek help in understanding what Hoosick Falls could learn from the West Virginia case. But he hesitated in doing so. The only "man of science" he knew was the town doctor, Marcus Martinez, a close family friend a few years older than he was, but Michael didn't want to bring his suspicions to Martinez until he thought he had more to go on.

During the time when Michael was advising his father on which course of kidney cancer treatment to choose, he had badgered Martinez so relentlessly with questions that he was now reluctant to raise an alarm before he felt he knew more. So, with not much more of a science background than an ability to click through articles while sitting at his computer, before raising what he suspected was the cause of Hoosick Falls's "bad luck" with his doctor friend and to village officials, Michael dedicated himself to learning what he could.

The scientific panel underwritten by the DuPont settlement was a good starting point. The epidemiologists considered a range of diseases and medical conditions. Although ruling out some diseases as being linked to PFOA, they concluded that there was a probable connection between the synthetic chemical and a list of terrible health outcomes. The scientists found that the long-term presence of PFOA in the West Virginia town's water was likely related to abnormal rates of testicular cancer, thyroid disease, ulcerative colitis, and hormone system disruption while also inducing higher levels of cholesterol, hypertension in pregnant women, and—most significant to Michael at the time—kidney cancer.[23]

While West Virginia's abnormal cluster of disease was apparently tied to PFOA in the water, there was still a missing element before Hoosick Falls's illness mystery could be solved. Although those same diseases had been found in the village at rates many found alarming, it still needed to be shown that the level of PFOA contamination in Hoosick Falls's water was significant enough to have caused these maladies.

Merely stating that Teflon was being produced and there were some number of people with these medical conditions was not enough. Despite wanting a definitive answer to the cause of his father's death, Michael didn't rule out the possibility that the presence of Teflon factories in Hoosick Falls and his father's disease was a coincidence that would not prove causality. He would have to connect the dots.

Michael also came to see that not everyone shared his interest in getting this story out, even some of those whose lives and whose families were most directly affected. At a family gathering a few weeks after he began his research, Michael shared what he had learned and his thinking that his father's death might somehow be related to chemicals used in the manufacture of Teflon, a product known to every adult in Hoosick Falls—whether they worked at a local factory or not. A family member cautioned him to be very careful before speaking publicly about his suspicions. "You don't go around making wild accusations like this unless you are sure," he was told. The repercussions could be severe.

The Norwegian playwright Henrik Ibsen's *An Enemy of the People* tells the story of a small Scandinavian town whose economic success is tied to the belief that there was a curative power in its water. Travelers came from near and far, and the town's prosperity grew with them. Then, Dr. Stockmann, a scientist and town resident, discovered that not only did the spa not have any positive health effect, but that the water was unsafe. If revealed, his information would lead to many in the town losing their financial investment in the local spa. He was urged to stay silent about what he had learned, which, after much soul-searching, he refused to do. Instead of his effort to care for the well-being of the townspeople and their visitors being appreciated, Dr. Stockmann became the "enemy of the people" that gave the 1882 play its name.

Michael didn't suffer the abuse that the fictional Dr. Stockmann does at the play's end, but his relative's admonition to not make unfounded accusations finally caused him to not take this on all by himself. Seeking to protect himself from being ostracized in the small town, he finally reached out to his friend, Marcus Martinez, the town doctor. Michael walked Martinez through what he had learned from his reading. The doctor agreed to take a look at the reports. Martinez called back a few weeks later and said he agreed that there might be something to what Michael feared was happening. The two of them decided to bring the news to the mayor, someone—not surprisingly—they both knew well.

As Michael recalled in an interview, the response of Dave Borge, Hoosick Falls's mayor, was akin to that of the mayor in *An Enemy of the People*. Borge told them that it wouldn't be necessary to notify everyone in the town. And when Michael suggested that the mayor quietly reach out to state and federal officials about these suspicions, Borge, a retired state employee, rejected the idea. The mayor even overruled Michael's proposal for them to test the village's water, as, he said, it would be a waste of money.

When Michael asked what the mayor thought should be done, Borge told them that it would be best for them to calm down. Hoosick Falls's population had finally stabilized in 2010 at about 3,500 people after decades of slow attrition from a post–World War II peak of 7,000. During periods of full employment, as many as 650 people were working in the town's Teflon factories. Helping them to keep their jobs and keeping everyone docile seemed to be more on the mayor's mind than a possible threat of tainted water.

Martinez pushed to have the information released, as it could be affecting people's health, and says he told Borge that the public had a right to know. In response to the entreaties by the two, Michael recalls Borge concluding the conversation by saying, "We have so many good things going on in Hoosick Falls. We're on our way back. Why would you want to get people all riled up and drive down property values and chase away the factories we still have?"

Efforts by phone and email to reach Borge for confirmation of the conversation were unsuccessful, but Martinez confirmed the contours of the conversation. "Borge definitely wanted to downplay the severity of the situation," Martinez says.[24] Dave Engel, a prominent environmental lawyer in Albany who later became the village's lawyer, also said that the conversation was consistent with what Borge said to him on several occasions, even long after the scientific evidence about PFOA contamination in Hoosick Falls's drinking water was beyond question.[25]

In the days that followed, in September 2014, Michael took matters into his own hands, and decided to get the water analyzed, even if he would have to pay for the tests himself. With a quick internet search, he found a company in Canada that tested for PFOA for a few hundred dollars. He was given instructions on how to get samples of the water and how to ship it. Michael sent the samples off to Canada, and waited for the results.

A Frequently Shifting EPA "Safe" Threshold

Within a few weeks of submitting the samples, the lab test results confirmed Michael's worst fears. The PFOA found in the tap water in his parents' home was more than double the EPA's then-safe threshold. In the tap water in his own home, where he lived with his wife and young son, the PFOA contamination was nearly triple that EPA level. Other local samples he had obtained and had sent for testing were also elevated.

Michael had connected the dots. Hoosick Falls had a drinking water contamination problem. People were getting sick with cancer and other illnesses tied to PFOA. Now something would need to be done. But when the issue was raised anew by Michael and his friend in October 2014, this time with proof in hand, the mayor suggested that the two of them think of the good of Hoosick Falls and not take their concerns any further. Even after news of the PFOA contamination became widely known, Borge would continue to express the belief that, as Martinez recalled it, there was no benefit to "making a spectacle." Remarkably, as late as December 2015, following the EPA's regional administrator, Judith Enck, sending a letter to the mayor saying the town's water was unsafe for drinking or cooking, and that information to the contrary on the town's website was incorrect, Borge continued to tell residents of Hoosick Falls that the decision on whether to consume local tap water was "a personal choice."[26]

That Michael figured out that there was PFOA in the town's water at all is extraordinary, and not just because he paid to have the tests done with his own money. Of the tens of thousands of chemicals in commerce in the U.S., fewer than one hundred drinking water contaminants are on a list of those regulated by the EPA, and PFOA isn't one of them. The EPA has a second list—capped by law at thirty suspected, but unregulated, drinking water contaminants—that the EPA is permitted to require testing for in any five-year period. PFOA was on that list from 2013 to 2015. While water utilities are obliged to test for and bring down the concentration of *regulated* contaminants to a level the EPA deems below a threat to human health, they have no obligation to routinely screen for, much less to treat, any of the contaminants on the list of thirty. All that the utilities are required to do is to periodically monitor the drinking water for each of the thirty for a few years and report what they find. Even if one of the suspect contaminants is discovered, there is no obligation to remove it from the drinking water or to continue to test for it. By federal law, the testing may only be used to gather information and isn't used to require any water utility to take action, even if the EPA could—but never has—later list it as a regulated contaminant.[27]

As confounding as this policy may be, small towns like Hoosick Falls have even less opportunity to discover a significant contamination of their drinking water. Under federal regulation, small towns are exempt from even the modest testing required of larger cities for unregulated, but suspect, contaminants.[28] This exemption was intended as a gift to the budgets of communities of ten thousand and fewer residents, but it is a gift that—as in Hoosick Falls—can come with consequences to public health. Because the EPA exemption is applied universally, even small towns that should be on high alert for PFOA or other chemicals have no obligation to test for any of the thirty suspected, but unregulated, contaminants. The EPA conducts a random screening of approximately 2 percent of water utilities in small towns, but not necessarily those most likely to be at risk.[29]

Until the crisis in Hoosick Falls was disclosed, because of its small population and the EPA exemption, its water was never tested for PFOA, even during its annual, federally mandated general water-quality assessments. It would seem like common sense to have such screenings in communities in which manufacturers are present and using such contaminants, whether the contaminants are regulated or not. Moreover, while lower-income communities and towns with declining populations are vulnerable on many levels, the lack of full-time advocates such as public officials or community organizations focusing on environmental or public health risks in drinking water, or otherwise, is part of that cycle of vulnerability.

There are many U.S. towns where Teflon and Teflon-related chemicals were mixed, used, disposed of, or utilized in manufacturing.[30] It might have been wise, especially after the initial discovery in Parkersburg, West Virginia, in 1999, for the EPA to have issued a rule to require testing for PFOA in every one of those locations, regardless of size. Similarly, there are other bedeviling contaminants that are still unregulated and which are likely to be found in places where they are either manufactured or used in manufacturing that would benefit from special screening. But no such rule exists to help protect any of these hundreds or thousands of places and, likely, in the aggregate, millions of Americans. This gap leaves it to a special citizen—a Paul Revere of sorts—to discover the threat and to raise the alarm to warn those nearby.

After Michael got confirmation of the elevated PFOA levels in his town, he was able to get many in Hoosick Falls to share his concerns, and to demand action. Strangely, though, even with PFOA contamination proven to be everywhere, the mayor was still eager to keep things calm and quiet. In late 2015, the corporations that owned the factories where PFOA was used—Honeywell and Saint-Gobain, both multibillion-dollar international companies—negotiated a deal with the mayor and village board that would cap the companies' liability with a payment of

$850,000.[31] More than half of that money would go to lawyers and a public relations firm, leaving the people of Hoosick Falls with a relative pittance to address current and future problems caused by the contamination.[32]

Hoosick Falls might have been stuck with the one-sided deal except that Dave Engel, the environmental lawyer from Albany then representing a group of dissidents from the town, shared the local PFOA story with a writer at the *Albany Times Union,* the largest newspaper in the area. It is also the newspaper sure to be read in the state capital. The journalist, Brendan Lyons, was a reporter and editor who covered environmental stories from time to time. As valuable as it always is to get friendly media to help alert others as to the presence of a life-threatening drinking water contaminant, it was the dissidents' special good fortune that Lyons's comprehensive coverage began appearing at the end of 2015. This coincided with Flint, Michigan's, water problems gaining a national audience that soon grew to be among the hottest news stories in the country.[33] The Flint story also showed that politicians who ignored drinking water contamination were at risk of ending their careers in public life, or even of facing criminal prosecution. Whether Hoosick Falls would be a New York State version of Flint was then still to be seen, but in the uproar that followed, the obviously-too-cheap deal between the companies and the town was killed.

Until Lyons's articles began making the front page in the state capital's newspaper, state officials, including those in the state's health and environment departments, had shown little interest in addressing the drinking water problem in Hoosick Falls. Their first reaction—similar to Flint and, sadly, elsewhere—was to say that the water was safe.[34] That continued to be the message of those high-ranking officials until it became politically too dangerous to continue with that claim.[35]

The change in approach by the state was caused by both local and federal pressure. After more than a year of telling everyone in Hoosick Falls that the water was safe, the mayor's credibility suffered irreparably when Lyons reported that the mayor, along with the law firm and public relations advisor that Hoosick Falls's village board had retained, were in close coordination with Saint-Gobain.[36] "The polluter and the mayor were secretly working together," said Lyons, "and this got everyone's attention."[37]

The EPA also caused New York State officials to pick up the speed of their response. For some time, the EPA had said the "safe" threshold of PFOA was 200 parts per trillion, a number far exceeded in both John and Michael Hickey's homes. But then the Hoosick Falls story began being covered in national media.[38] Soon thereafter, the EPA issued a new guideline cutting the number in half to 100 parts per trillion, and then within a few months, lowering it yet further to 70 parts per trillion. The science may have changed, but not likely so much or so fast. Fear of embarrassment may have played a role, with a possible lesson that the EPA's contaminant danger thresholds can be politically influenced.

But even the EPA's current lower limit at 70 parts per trillion may be the wrong level. One respected professor of public health, Harvard's Philippe Grandjean, believes that a PFOA threshold of even one part per trillion may be a threat to pregnant women, their fetuses, and also to young children.[39] To add to the confusion, the federal Agency for Toxic Substances and Disease Registry, a branch of the U.S. Centers for Disease Control and Prevention, more recently issued a report proposing that the maximum safe level for PFOA in water should be at 11 parts per trillion.[40] At any of these supposedly safe PFOA thresholds, the PFOA levels in the homes of John Hickey (440 parts per trillion) and Michael Hickey (580 parts per trillion) far exceeded every one of them.

Whatever the correct number, it is hard to not want to avert your eyes from the Hoosick Falls story. With a few simple measures, so much misery and heartache could almost certainly have been prevented. Hoosick Falls and many other places across the U.S. have compromised drinking water, and people in those places have no idea why their young neighbor is getting cancer, or why their child has developed one of several hormonal disruptions. While filtration methods differ for different contaminants, PFOA can be easily removed from drinking water with a system called granular activated carbon, or GAC, whereby the PFOA becomes attached to small granules of charcoal in a filter. That GAC has been available as a treatment technique for drinking water since long before Teflon production first came to Hoosick Falls makes the likely PFOA-inflicted misery in the town all the more tragic.[41]

In October 2017, a GAC system was installed in the Hoosick Falls central drinking water facility and in the basements of all homes in surrounding areas that get PFOA-contaminated water from other groundwater sources like private wells.[42] The state government has said it will pursue Honeywell and Saint-Gobain for reimbursement. If so, it is believed that when all is done, the corporations will be held responsible for at least $25 million, many multiples of their almost accepted original offer.

Thanks to the universal use of GAC filters in Hoosick Falls, the town's drinking water now has no amount of detectable PFOA, making the water now free of that contaminant. But for many in the town, and even for many others who grew up there but have moved away, the change will have come too late.

Two months after the town doctor, Marcus Martinez, then forty-two, gave Michael Hickey his view that it was a good idea to test the water, he became ill and was soon diagnosed with cancer, leading to a series of surgeries and rounds of chemotherapy. And as word about Hoosick Falls's water has spread, people who left the town after high school or college—people now in their twenties and thirties—have gotten in touch with Michael Hickey to report the onset of medical maladies, including ulcerative colitis, thyroid disease, and testicular cancer, all identified by researchers as potential effects of drinking PFOA-contaminated water.[43] Whether all, some, or none of these were caused by the town's drinking water is impossible to say with absolute certainty, but it is, likewise, impossible to know what future diseases or birth defects might lurk in the bodies of the people of Hoosick Falls. Yet, here, too, the low-key Michael Hickey is trying to make a difference.

Some people in Hoosick Falls have joined together in a class action lawsuit against Honeywell and Saint-Gobain for the drop in the value of their homes. Michael declined to join that lawsuit, saying that he isn't planning on leaving Hoosick Falls anytime soon and that, anyway, he doesn't want to look like he's in this for financial gain. While refusing to be part of that litigation, Michael is the lead plaintiff in a suit widely joined by his fellow townspeople asking for medical monitoring expenses to be covered by Honeywell and Saint-Gobain. While many of these diseases and medical problems can't be prevented, early detection can get possibly lifesaving treatment to people long exposed to high doses of PFOA.

"We are now all at risk of cancers and thyroid disease, and other frightening illnesses," says Michael Hickey. "None of this is because of any fault of our own. We just drank the water."

Two

THE EPA TAKES CONTROL OF DRINKING WATER

*"The feeling in the early years of the EPA was that the agency was
here to save the world. . . . Everybody thought we were on a mission
to protect public health and the environment. Over time,
that feeling went away."*
—Jim Elder, former director of the EPA Office
of Ground Water and Drinking Water

M ICHAEL HICKEY WASN'T the only son motivated to address water problems after his father died a premature and painful death from contaminated water. There was another one who also did so, and with great consequence. Both sons stood up for what they believed was right. Both sons were at odds with the conventional wisdom of their day. And, more than a hundred years apart, both sons were ultimately vindicated. But unlike Michael Hickey, whose influence may never travel much beyond his village's borders, this other son has touched the lives of billions and, no doubt, has saved the lives of millions.

When the American Civil War broke out, John Rose Leal left his wife and their then-six-year-old son—John Laing Leal—and his rural medical practice a few hours north of New York City to enlist with the Union forces. He was appointed as doctor for a New York regiment.

Wounded twice in combat, Leal became permanently disabled when Confederate forces surrounded his regiment on a barrier island near Charleston, South Carolina. During that May 1863 siege, Leal and nearly all of the men in the regiment became sick with dysentery after drinking tainted water. Several of them died. Leal survived the war and returned to the practice of medicine, but, due to acute gastrointestinal ailments caused by the dysentery, he could no longer travel long distances on horseback to visit patients. To accommodate his infirmity, the family moved to Paterson, New Jersey, where John Rose Leal's urban clinic spared him the need to travel.[1]

After finishing college, Leal's son, John Laing Leal, decided to follow his father's career path, and to also become a doctor. As was the practice then, in addition to classroom study, medical students served as interns to experienced physicians. John Laing Leal had the benefit of interning for his father. But in August 1882, during the son's third year of medical studies, his father died following an agonizing episode of complications from the waterborne disease that had continuously plagued him since his military service.

After graduation from medical school, the younger Leal set up a practice in New Jersey, and, while busy with that and a family of his own, soon became fascinated with the relatively new and evolving world of microbiology. He also became active in what would today be called public health and epidemiology, learning what he could about the causes of—and ways of stopping—epidemics.

In 1897, following an outbreak of typhoid fever in Maidstone, England, and knowing of the purifying effect of chlorine, the local reservoir there was treated with a large dose of the chemical. It was the first time that chemicals had been used to neutralize bacteria in a community's drinking water.[2] Until the Maidstone reservoir was chlorinated, the conventional wisdom—itself only a few decades old—had been that the best way of keeping people safe from getting sick from their drinking water was to obtain water resources upstream of where human and animal waste was discharged.

By the late nineteenth century, major cities around the world began the costly effort of building sewers to divert that waste away from the upstream parts of the rivers from where those cities got their water. With these new, expensive sewer systems in place, although epidemics did not come to an end, the number and intensity of them significantly declined.[3] Due to this success, and also due to the large sunk cost in having built those sewers, there was little interest in exploring new techniques or spending public funds to try to find yet safer drinking water.

Nonetheless, Maidstone's use of chlorine got Leal thinking. While Maidstone added a large amount of the chemical *following* the start of its local epidemic, Leal began wondering if the addition of small and ongoing quantities of chlorine *before* water was pumped to people's homes might be a boon to public health. He soon had an opportunity to act on his hunch.

In 1902, Leal was hired as the sanitary advisor to the Jersey City Water Supply Company, a privately owned company that supplied the city's water.[4] Jersey City, then (and now) New Jersey's largest city after Newark, had a population of a little more than 200,000 and was one of the twenty most populous cities in the U.S. Without notice to the people of Jersey City or its government, Leal began a series of experiments in which he sought the precise amount of chlorine needed to kill waterborne bacteria. Aside from effectiveness in killing pathogens, which he could have achieved with high volumes of chlorine, Leal also wanted those drinking the water to not be able to smell or taste the presence of chlorine. After six years, he believed he found the perfect balance, and, in his capacity as sanitary advisor to the city's water supplier, began adding small amounts of chlorine to Jersey City's drinking water. It was the first time that a chemical had been added to drinking water on a preventive basis, and not in response to an epidemic.

When it was discovered that Leal had put chlorine into Jersey City's drinking water supply without public notice or discussion, his actions provoked outrage. He was accused of poisoning the water supply.[5]

Leal and his employer, the Jersey City Water Supply Company, were sued by the city.

A long and highly publicized trial pitted some of the best scientific and technical minds of the day against Leal and his codefendants. Due to the renown of several witnesses testifying against Leal and his practices, and also the sensationalized idea that the doctor might be poisoning the population of a major city, the trial was followed beyond Jersey City.[6] But Leal's arguments won the day. His unrebutted demonstration that total bacteria concentrations dropped from 30,000 to 40,000 per milliliter* to six to eight per milliliter after filtration and chlorination was persuasive to the judge who conducted the trial without a jury. In his ruling, the trial judge exonerated Leal and the others, and concluded that the Jersey City Water Supply Company could keep its contract supplying water to the city and would be permitted to continue adding chlorine to the community's water supply.[7]

The November 1910 decision in that Jersey City courtroom had implications near and far, and long into the future. Unsurprisingly, with the addition of chlorine in Jersey City's water, deaths from typhoid and other waterborne diseases dropped to near zero.[8] Within ten years, more than one thousand U.S. cities and towns—equaling 75 percent of all those on a municipal water grid—were using chlorination to safeguard their drinking water. By 1926, 3,200 U.S. communities, and nearly 100 percent of those getting water other than from private wells, were having their drinking water treated with some dosage of chlorine in one form or another.[9] The use of chlorine to disinfect drinking water was adopted as an inexpensive way to improve public health.

Chlorination of drinking water is now the norm worldwide. As a result, major outbreaks of fatal disease from waterborne microorganisms are very unusual in all but the most desperately deprived nations.[10] But the Chlorine Revolution came with a price beyond the relatively small cost of building the treatment facilities and purchasing the chemical.

---

* There are nearly five milliliters in a teaspoon.

Prior to Leal and his chlorine treatment of water, there was consensus that sources of drinking water had to be kept as pristine as possible. Because water was drawn from places upriver, there was recognition that communities needed to protect those sources from factories or industrial development that produced contaminants or from clusters of homes generating sewage, all of which could get into the downriver water supply.[11]

With the extraordinary effectiveness of chlorine and other related chemicals, however, it became harder to resist pressure from business interests and to justify saying no to industrial and residential expansion. Mayors were happy with the expanded tax base these new homes and factories provided, and following adoption of chemical water treatment, they had a convenient excuse to move ahead with economic development near sources of drinking water. It also allowed them to spend minimally on source water protection, if anything was spent at all. With chlorine lulling communities into a false sense of complacency, source water around the U.S. became widely, and inevitably, polluted.

The second major effect of the addition of chlorine wasn't detected until the early 1970s, more than sixty years after Leal first added chlorine to Jersey City's water. Scientists came to realize that chlorine and other disinfectants added to water were, at times, causing a previously undetected chemical reaction. When chlorine mixed with naturally occurring organic material such as the residue of dead leaves that had fallen or been blown into water sources, chemicals called trihalomethanes, or THMs, were created. While the chemical reaction between chlorine and decomposing organic material hadn't previously been known, THMs had already been shown to cause cancer in laboratory animals and was suspected—and later confirmed—as being a possible human carcinogen.

With national concern about the safety of drinking water then driven by persistent media reports about toxic matter getting into tap water, especially in communities along the Mississippi River, news that chlorine might be causing a health hazard instantly became a major story.[12]

After all, if people knew anything about their drinking water, it was that chlorine was supposed to be keeping it safe—and not, as was now reported, putting them and their children at risk. For an alarmed public, this new worry about waterborne dangers from what came to be called "disinfection by-products" provided the final push for Congress to begin to make safe drinking water a subject for major legislation and for oversight by the EPA.

Had it not been for John Laing Leal and his insight that chlorine might end the terror of periodic epidemics, drinking water might still be seen as a conveyance for harmful bacteria. But now, also thanks to Leal, even if less directly, the safety and healthfulness of drinking water in the U.S. would have an opportunity to significantly improve again.

In December 1974, spurred by the drumbeat of news stories about the safety of chlorinated drinking water, the Safe Drinking Water Act was passed, and signed into law by President Gerald Ford.[13]

Water Utilities and Public Health

The Safe Drinking Water Act had first been introduced in 1970. Even with the heightened awareness of environmental issues of that year, culminating in the first Earth Day, the proposed bill failed to get the necessary support. It failed again when it was proposed anew in 1972. Lobbying by many mayors and heads of water utilities kept the two earlier versions of the bill from even coming up for a vote. These water utility executives and local officials saw the proposed law as a burden, and their concerns were passed along to their local member of Congress. With no organized constituency making demands for better drinking water, both Democrats and Republicans agreed to bottle up the bill—at least until media and public pressure following the chlorine-THM discovery became too great to put off a vote.[14]

With the 1974 drinking water legislation, Congress gave specific tasks to the EPA, to the states, and to the local water utilities.[15] The new law made the still young EPA the senior partner in this three-way, federal-state-local water relationship, but with opportunities for significant roles for each.

Of greatest urgency to Congress at that time, the EPA was directed to solve the chlorine problem, and to give the public confidence that the disinfection by-products cancer scare was under control. At the same time, the authors of the bill wanted the EPA to identify what was assumed would be a growing list of industrial and other contaminants in drinking water, and to give guidance on how to protect the public from them. In turn, the law put specific obligations upon states to supervise water utilities and made the utilities responsible for monitoring those contaminants identified by the EPA. Once those contaminants were discovered in drinking water, utilities were obliged to neutralize, control, or eliminate the pollutants identified by the EPA.

Although the Safe Drinking Water Act permits states to set standards higher (but not lower) than those of the EPA in contaminant control, most of what is asked of the states is administrative.[16] For example, each state is responsible for collecting EPA-required data from its local water utilities and forwarding the data at regular intervals to the federal agency. Except in very rare circumstances when the EPA may choose to step in, if a local water provider violates the Safe Drinking Water Act, or regulations under it, and has to be disciplined, it is the state's responsibility to do it. In practice, state government officials are often reluctant to get into a dispute with a local water utility, and this has been an impediment to enforcement.

Completing this governance triangle created by Congress, the water utility or the local municipal government that served as the water provider was made responsible for making sure that all of the EPA's regulations were implemented. The utility was required to monitor the local water supply for a range of EPA-identified contaminants. If there was a failure to monitor the water properly, or if the water had contaminants above the permitted level, the local utility was obliged—in most cases pursuant to an under-enforced honor system—to report those violations.

These new obligations imposed on water utilities and local governments were soon unpopular, with complaints heard about Congress
compelling local expenditures without contribution from the federal
government.

Two years before the Safe Drinking Water Act was signed into law,
a bipartisan Congress passed the 1972 Clean Water Act by lopsided mar-
gins over the veto of President Richard Nixon. That law had as its goal
ending the dumping of untreated or inadequately treated sewage and
other waste into surface water such as lakes, rivers, and streams by factories, animal feedlots, and municipal wastewater treatment plants. What
made the Clean Water Act especially popular with Congress was that it
opened up the federal treasury to every community to help upgrade or,
in many cases, rebuild its wastewater treatment plant. Under the Clean
Water Act, the federal government agreed to cover 80 percent of the
local wastewater treatment project expense. Since everyone could participate in the bonanza, only the most determined budget deficit hawks
voted against it, and few did.[17]

The obligations and financial burdens that came along with the Clean
Water Act were accepted—at least, initially—as part of a good deal for
participating municipalities of every size. With the Safe Drinking Water
Act, though, it was all spinach and no candy. It had many requirements
and potential expenses for municipalities and water utilities, with nothing in return but the intangible value of cleaner, safer water for the public. While better water would seem to be benefit enough, for many of
those who provide that drinking water, it isn't—and that fact reveals an
important truth about many, if not most, of America's water utilities.

Public water utilities didn't, and still mostly don't, see themselves as
part of the community's public health infrastructure. This doesn't mean
they are engaged in nefarious deeds or eager to see anyone get sick, but
that, if better health outcomes are the goal, there is a misalignment
between the interests of utilities and the public. At the risk of over-
generalizing, utilities deliver water that is "good enough" at the lowest
cost possible. Working against that, expenses are driven up by regula-

tions and the need to purchase new equipment or technology. To reduce spending, many water utilities also defer maintenance and leave pipes in the ground long past their useful life. Further, as most water utilities are responsive to mayors, the utilities do what they can to make them happy by keeping water charges as low as possible. Mayors know that voters see water fees as a kind of tax, and without a reason to have to pay more, consumers will always prefer lower prices. As a result, rather than providing the best water possible, utilities end up providing that "good enough" water, with "good" being defined by what is minimally demanded by the EPA and its state counterparts. There are, of course, exceptions, but this is the norm.

To the chagrin of many of those utilities, the Safe Drinking Water Act created a structure that changed the way water was managed and regulated in the U.S. Before the law's passage, that regulation and management had always been under the near-exclusive control of the states and local governments. For better or worse, the water utilities and those government bodies knew how to work with each other to their mutual benefit, even if not always resulting in providing the purest water possible.

With the EPA being given the authority by the Safe Drinking Water Act to set maximum allowable levels in the drinking water for every contaminant it chose to regulate, utilities—which had tried to stymie the passage of the law—would now have that same interest in keeping regulated contaminants to a minimum. And when they couldn't stop a contaminant from getting on the EPA list of chemicals that had to be screened, then utilities would have an incentive to have the threshold for acceptable contamination set as high as possible, thereby making the utility's treatment costs as low as possible. Strangely, rather than resisting this effort to keep the Safe Drinking Water Act from leading to the best drinking water possible, the EPA was mostly willing to oblige the utilities' wish for minimal enforcement.

The EPA Moves Slowly

It didn't take long for Congress to grow dissatisfied with what turned out to be the EPA's slow-paced hunt for contaminants and the setting of standards for each of them. In 1974, in the aftermath of the Watergate scandal, the "throw the bums out" sentiment led to many new faces in Congress following the off-year federal elections. One of those elected in the Class of '74 was Henry Waxman, a passionate California liberal, then thirty-five years old, representing Beverly Hills. The new congressman had begun concentrating his legislative interests on health and the environment when elected to the California legislature six years earlier, and he continued this effort with his election to the House of Representatives.

"I arrived [in January 1975] at the start of a changing era," Waxman, who retired from his long career in Congress in 2015, said in an interview. "The young Democrats who came in with me arrived with an agenda to shake the place up." Waxman ended up chairing a subcommittee with direct oversight of the EPA and its approach to protecting drinking water.[18]

With thousands of new compounds being added to the national chemical inventory each year, members of Congress like Henry Waxman became frustrated with the EPA and its slow pace in using its new powers to identify and regulate potentially hazardous contaminants getting into drinking water. The failure to act at that time wasn't, the thinking went, only because of water industry efforts to block specific actions by the EPA, but also because of the agency's own painstaking, overly bureaucratic style. Indeed, the water utilities, and their allies, had enormous political clout that they were prepared to use when necessary, but the EPA had also fallen far short, Waxman and others said, of what it needed to be doing to protect the country's drinking water.

Was the criticism fair? Had—and has—the EPA failed to seize the opportunity to improve drinking water quality and safety?

Opinions about the EPA and its effectiveness in ensuring safe drinking water are akin to a Rorschach test. What you see in the agency drinking water efforts tends to reflect whether you believe the EPA's primary responsibility should be centered on public health or whether economic growth should be an equal or greater concern. The EPA has certainly evolved over time, but there is little doubt that the perceived halo around the organization has endured, at least in the progressive imagination. When most of those who like the idea of government playing a larger role in our lives think about federal agencies effectively looking out for our well-being, the EPA is likely to be a contender for a top prize.

But some insiders say the reputation—at least as regards drinking water—isn't deserved, and not just because, from time to time, anti-regulation EPA administrators serve as the agency's chief. For some with years of EPA experience, it is a bipartisan failure. Administrations come and go, and with them political appointees, but the permanent bureaucracy of the EPA never seems to make a big leap forward in identifying and regulating new contaminants in drinking water.

Jim Elder, a career EPA official who ended his EPA tenure serving as the head of the agency's Office of Ground Water and Drinking Water, joined the organization in 1971, months after the environmental agency was formed in December 1970. "The feeling in the early years of the EPA," he says, "was that the agency was here to save the world, starting with the U.S. When the agency was young, everybody thought we were on a mission to protect public health and the environment. Over time, that feeling went away. Starting in the 1980s, and with only a few exceptions since, the agency got stuck in an endless process of analysis and cost-benefit calculations."[19]

One prominent environmental activist, Erik Olson, who has long paid special attention to drinking water issues and who worked at the EPA early in his career, believes that the EPA's bureaucratic style is "overwhelmingly a result of political opposition, and water utility and other industry pushback." Olson refers to the EPA's relationship with the drinking water industry as "almost a Stockholm Syndrome," a psychological situation in which a captive comes to profess the outlook of the captor.

The problem, he thinks, is less bureaucratic impasse and more a response to pressure.[20]

An equally harsh view of opportunities presented and lost is expressed by Ronnie Levin, a thirty-seven-year veteran of policy analysis at the EPA who is now at the Harvard School of Public Health. "There are many very smart, caring people at the EPA," she says. "The problem is that, in the case of the [EPA's] Water Office, regardless of the administration or the party in power, the work of the agency is dominated by industry. The AWWA," the acronym for the American Water Works Association, "is really the one that calls the shots. Water utilities aren't public health agencies, and the AWWA is analogous to the American Petroleum Institute and other strong industry groups. It should be seen as such." In bolstering her point about the EPA's propensity to be overly solicitous of industry associations, Levin adds that in the regulation of pesticides, the chemical and agriculture industry groups have a similar influence at the EPA.[21]

A more balanced view is offered by a former senior EPA water official, an appointee during a Democratic administration. His current employer won't permit him to be quoted by name or to reveal what position he had at the EPA, but, speaking not for attribution, he acknowledges that the EPA could do more. Even so, he is quick to point out that the EPA has limits on what can be realistically achieved without a change in funding—and, by implication, mandate—from Congress.

"What is it that [government] water people care about?" he asks rhetorically. "We care about clean water generally and have many people working on different kinds of potentially dangerous things in the water like lead or disinfection by-products. But we also have to be realistic. We get limited resources and that causes us to put a lot of effort into trying to implement the rules already on the books. Because of that, we put our energy into what can kill people quickly, like microbes in the water." That, he says, can make it "tough to focus on 'new' contaminants that may hurt or kill you more slowly, especially where the science is uncertain or evolving."[22]

For the then-recently-elected Henry Waxman looking at drinking water issues in the 1970s, that lack of focus on "new" contaminants was unacceptable. Utilizing the power that came to him with his chairmanship of a subcommittee responsible for oversight of drinking water policy, Waxman was determined to light a fire under the EPA. Even if the science was "uncertain or evolving," Waxman wanted more action, and he thought he knew how to go about getting it.

"The Clean Air Act was passed in 1970 before I got to Congress," Waxman says. "But the reason it was already producing results by the early 1980s was that it sought controls and set standards above what was then believed possible. Without goals, we'd never have gotten cleaner air. I was convinced we'd never get safer drinking water without pushing the EPA, the states, and the utilities to reach higher."

Waxman's goal was to have all potential contaminants under review, or at least as many as possible. He also wanted a standard to be developed for these potentially dangerous contaminants at a level of protection above what normal, healthy adults could tolerate. "Standards should be set for the most vulnerable," Waxman says. "Children, elderly, and the immunosuppressed have an even harder time with contaminants than healthy adults do," and it was for these vulnerable populations that Waxman wanted to have the EPA contaminant standards set.[23]

The Safe Drinking Water Act Is Amended (Part 1)

For advocates of safe drinking water and a faster-moving EPA like Waxman, what was initially cause for despair turned into a victory. In 1980, Ronald Reagan was elected president. He appointed Anne Gorsuch (mother of current U.S. Supreme Court Justice Neil Gorsuch) to head the EPA and James Watt as secretary of the interior. Both were clumsy politically and inept as administrators. Worse, they both underestimated the degree to which Americans had come to appreciate the environmental safeguards that promised to provide cleaner air and water.

The pair's much publicized comments about plans to cut regulation ran into a buzz saw of opposition. Despite their bluster about reducing the government's footprint in the environmental arena, neither Gorsuch nor Watt succeeded in cutting very much in their respective areas of control. In an example of unintended consequences, by their threats to cut regulations and their open disregard for enforcement of existing ones, they managed to get public interest groups motivated to demand yet more environmental regulation.[24]

Waxman saw an opportunity. Working with a number of environmentally-minded, moderate Republicans, Congress came together to push back on the Reagan administration's plan to cut regulations.[25] Among other actions, they decided to put significant demands on the EPA to move more quickly on identifying and regulating new contaminants in drinking water. And fearful of a future EPA chief like Anne Gorsuch who might sabotage their goals, they wanted to remove any flexibility that the agency might have then or in the future in delaying their new approach.[26]

Ironically, had it not been for Reagan's appointment of Gorsuch and Watt, it is likely that those environmental groups would not have seen an infusion of cash, energy, and new members. Without it, even with Waxman's passion for the issue, it is possible that the lethargic pace of water regulation might have continued, or even slowed, due to bureaucratic inertia.

Despite great expectations of what the Safe Drinking Water Act would deliver, in the twelve years following its passage in 1974, only twenty-three contaminants had been regulated, and not all of them were chemicals.[27] But now, with key people from both parties in Congress sensitized to the issue—along with a new generation of well-funded environmental organizations to lead on ideas and advocacy, and a nation of outraged people who wanted more, not less, protection for clean air and clean water—the moment was primed for action.

The activists in Congress used the momentum they had to reconceive the Safe Drinking Water Act. With changes that came to be known as the 1986 Amendments, the law was significantly overhauled. Creating great new goals for the EPA, the changed law prescribed a sense of urgency at the agency. If it took from 1974 to 1986 for the EPA to regulate twenty-three contaminants, now Congress was demanding that the EPA set standards for no fewer than eighty-three chemical and other contaminants in just the following three years. These eighty-three contaminants were taken from a list that the EPA's own staff scientists had suggested be regulated but which the White House Office of Management and Budget (OMB) had blocked due to economic concerns.[28] The only flexibility Congress offered the EPA was an authorization for the agency to substitute up to seven contaminants in place of those on Congress's list of eighty-three contaminants, but only if the agency believed that any of substituted compounds posed a greater health threat.[29]

There was yet more.

To demonstrate that a permanent change of culture was expected at the EPA, Congress further insisted that the EPA's hunt for drinking water contaminants would continue when those initial eighty-three contaminants were regulated in 1989. As soon as that large task was done, Congress wanted the EPA to select and regulate an additional twenty-five drinking water contaminants by 1991. And continuing with this upbeat tempo, Congress made it obligatory that after the 1991 results, the EPA would have to choose and regulate another twenty-five contaminants every three years thereafter.[30] As if all of that wasn't enough, Congress also used the 1986 legislation to set a new standard for the amount of lead permitted in pipes, taking away from the EPA its usual role in being the government entity to set those standards.[31]

For members of Congress, like Henry Waxman, this was, he then thought, a crowning achievement.[32] Given the large, veto-proof majority in favor of the 1986 Amendments, even Ronald Reagan—who had appointed Anne Gorsuch and James Watt, setting off the backlash that led to more protection for drinking water—agreed to sign the new law.

While taking some credit for it, as would any smart politician, Reagan used the signing ceremony as an opportunity to also offer some objections to the new version of the law, lamenting that it would take away much of the EPA's discretion on managing safe drinking water.[33]

The Safe Drinking Water Act Is Amended (Part 2)

Political winds can shift quickly. After getting broad-based support for aggressively regulating contaminants that might be in drinking water, sentiment began to change. According to polls, Americans' enthusiasm for better drinking water is highest when "someone else"—corporations or government—is paying, and this was true here, too.[34] Especially as it became clearer that better health standards for drinking water would come with new obligations for water utilities, the new health-protective approach soon had many active opponents.

In addition, the passage of the 1986 Amendments was seen as a great victory by leading environmental organizations. But following the success, many became complacent and moved their attention and funding to other areas of concern. With their guard dropped, antagonists of drinking water regulation moved to counterattack.

As demanded by the 1986 Amendments, the EPA was required to begin analyzing and setting standards for the eighty-three contaminants listed in the legislation. With the announcement of each new standard, the nation's water utilities were obliged to begin monitoring to assure that the local drinking water did not exceed the newly set maximum level of the contaminant. The utilities were given permission to do less monitoring if they could show that the regulated contaminant wasn't present at a dangerous level, but that didn't release them from the obligation to test from time to time to be sure conditions had not changed. A failure to miss the presence of a regulated contaminant in the future could, in principle, subject the utility to citations and fines.[35]

While the monitoring was a relatively small expense for large utilities because they could spread the costs of compliance over a large user base, operators of small water systems began complaining about the sudden imposition of new mandatory spending. These costs, they and other local officials argued, were a strain on tight budgets that were already competing for funding with education, police, roads, and other local concerns. Governors and mayors of both parties complained about the "unfunded mandates" that the legislation imposed, with these state and local officials saying that if the federal government wanted to compel activities to be carried out by the water utilities, Congress should pay for them.[36]

Building on these complaints, opponents of the 1986 Amendments found a way to turn the environmentalists' arguments against them. The opponents said that, by Congress compelling the EPA to regulate all eighty-three contaminants with equal urgency, the EPA was distracted from looking out for the public's welfare by not having the flexibility to prioritize its efforts on the greatest threats.[37] This position may have been sincere or contrived, but either way, opponents of the 1986 Amendments attempted to position themselves as being the true advocates of clean water and public health.

Compounding the problems for advocates of the 1986 Amendments, a series of U.S. General Accounting Office (now the Government Accountability Office) (GAO) studies reported widespread under-compliance and noncompliance with the new law. At all levels of government, the GAO revealed, the law wasn't being followed as written or as intended. Because of funding shortfalls, the report found, the EPA wouldn't be likely to complete the evaluation and regulation of the eighty-three contaminants on schedule. It also reported that water utilities around the country weren't testing newly regulated contaminants and reporting to the states as they were obliged to do, and the states were not following up with utilities that were not fully compliant.[38] Apparently, with no effective enforcement mechanism, many water utilities felt safe in ignoring inconvenient parts or costly requirements of the legislation.

The turning point came, however, with the 1994 congressional elections. Made famous by Newt Gingrich's Contract with America, the elections brought a Republican majority to the House of Representatives for the first time in forty years. The new members of Congress and their leaders were no less ideologically committed than the Democrats who had pushed for the enhancements in the Safe Drinking Water Act a decade earlier. Unlike their liberal colleagues, their philosophy drove them to undo much of the centralization of power in the federal government that had accumulated over many years. Among their targets was a rollback of the 1986 Amendments, if not the repeal of the entire Safe Drinking Water Act itself.

With the support of many water utilities, as well as the National Governors Association, the Conference of Mayors, and others, legislation was introduced that would eliminate mandatory standard setting by the EPA. Likewise, there would be no minimum number of contaminants to be regulated in every three-year cycle. The EPA would have the power to identify a drinking water contaminant and to set standards for it, but with an important caveat: For most standards, the benefits for the nation's health would have to be determined and balanced by the economic cost of that regulation.[39]

Although it sounded like common sense to look at both the benefit and the burden of regulating a contaminant, Henry Waxman, then still the leader in the House on drinking water safety, had long been opposed to that approach. "You can always measure the costs of environmental policy," Waxman says. "That's a relatively easy number to produce. But the benefits are harder to quantify. And of course, industry will always have a reason to overstate the cost."[40]

But Waxman and the other environmentalists in Congress were in retreat, and accepted that they would have to cut the best deal they could make. This would include accepting what became known as the cost-benefit methodology. The 1996 Amendments, as the second major overhaul of the Safe Drinking Water Act came to be called, reversed the goals of the 1986 Amendments and ended the effort to aggressively regulate contaminants. Even in retreat, Waxman and the others were able to get a few new benefits, even if, in practice, some of them proved to not have much value.

The new law incorporated ongoing efforts to identify and regulate potential carcinogens from disinfection by-products. Regulation and standard setting of maximum arsenic levels—a hot-button issue for members of Congress from states and districts with large natural deposits of it who opposed regulation—would be permitted. Local water utilities would be required to produce a report for their customers no less than annually describing the quality of the local water and listing the regulated contaminants found in it. And most popular, even among new Republicans in the House of Representatives from rural districts, a pot of money was created—about $600 million in the first year, with more promised to follow—to lend to public water utilities at favorable rates to help bring them up to higher standards.[41] The 1996 Amendments also authorized a limited amount of that fund for grants targeted at economically disadvantaged communities.

With the mandatory regulation of contaminants about to be ended, Waxman made one more push. He succeeded in getting agreement for ongoing EPA-led research on the potential presence of contaminants in drinking water, but, even so, the EPA was prohibited from studying more than thirty of them in any five-year period. To ease the burden on smaller water utilities, mandatory testing for the thirty contaminants was limited to the utilities serving large communities, with only about 2 percent of smaller water utilities, like the one in Hoosick Falls, being randomly tested.

These studies, though, were not to be unconstrained explorations into improving water quality. The 1996 Amendments explicitly required that the studies be utilized for the purpose of collecting data.[42] This investigation would create no immediate obligation to do anything about any contaminants found, even if Waxman's hope, as later shared by one of his senior staff members, was that their discovery would, at a minimum, lead to regulation, and, perhaps, encourage the public's return to demanding safer, contaminant-free drinking water.[43]

It would make sense, after all, that if a contaminant were found in the water—and it was a potential threat to public health—that a law named the Safe Drinking Water Act would provide the EPA with the means to protect the public, and that the EPA would do so as quickly as possible.

Unfortunately, it didn't quite work out that way.

Three

AN ENDLESS ROAD TO NOWHERE

*"While we are waiting for some perfect study
that tells us what to do, we are leaving
populations exposed to contaminants."*
—Dr. Melanie Marty,
Senior Scientist, California Office
of Health Hazard Assessment

T HE IMPLIED PROMISE of the Safe Drinking Water Act is twofold. First, that the EPA will identify contaminants in drinking water and, second, when found, it will promptly figure out how best to protect Americans from the health hazards those toxic substances present. If that is the expectation, the reality has been different. The EPA's search for contaminants in drinking water is slow paced and haphazard. And when contaminants are identified—often by independent researchers— there is no urgency by the EPA in setting standards so that water utilities will know how much of the toxic element to remove.

In examining the EPA's dysfunction on this (and much else), it is worth looking at the agency's role in the possible regulation of perchlorate, an industrial chemical. Long known to be a health hazard, perchlorate has been under EPA investigation for more than twenty years. Until a decision is made to regulate it, drinking water utilities have no obligation to remove it from water systems.[1] When, if ever, the EPA will come to a conclusion that is protective of public health is a question everyone should be asking, whether or not they are directly affected by this one contaminant.

Drinking water concerns tend to be local and personal, ordinarily limited to worries about one's immediate family and neighborhood. Yet, even if perchlorate isn't in your drinking water, there is still good reason to be concerned about the EPA's slow process in deciding what to do about it.

It shouldn't be a surprise that at the same time the EPA isn't regulating perchlorate, it also isn't actively pursuing other potential health hazards in drinking water either. As it goes with perchlorate, so it goes with another unregulated or under-regulated contaminant that may be in your water. The threat to public health—and to your health—comes as much from what the EPA isn't doing as from what comes from any contaminant that may be in drinking water. Without a culture change forced on the EPA, there is no reason that the agency will adopt a different tempo or a philosophy more protective of health. And without a new approach to drinking water at the EPA, as ever more chemicals are introduced into commerce, nearly everyone may be at risk.

While the focus throughout this book is on drinking water, in setting protective health standards, the EPA needs to look beyond drinking water as a medium for contamination. In its analysis, the agency must also take into account all likely routes of contamination for every suspect chemical that is or should be reviewed. This requires having the EPA measure the "multi-media" impact of those toxic elements to get a better sense of the true extent of the danger. Although each chemical is different, the risk from a drinking water contaminant can come from more than just the water that carries it. The same chemical can also be transmitted by the air we breathe, the food we eat, and even absorbed through contact with our skin.

In the case of perchlorate, an additional danger comes from fruit and vegetables that have been irrigated with contaminated water or washed with perchlorate-contaminated bleach. A person in, say, Florida who is drinking water containing perchlorate will have that exposure amplified by eating produce grown in California, if the water used for irrigation contained perchlorate. High levels of perchlorate have also been found by the FDA in a variety of other foods including, most concerningly, baby food.[2] The potential harm from the aggregate of these other sources of contamination argues for less complacency and more protective standards.

Strangely, given that the most severe effects of perchlorate are felt on fetuses and newborns, following the EPA's general approach to testing, the agency initially investigated the chemical's effect on healthy 170-pound males. Following a ferocious argument in Congress (not specifically related to perchlorate) as to whether testing should be required for the effect of drinking water contaminants on those most likely to be injured by them, a compromise was reached.

The 1996 Amendments to the Safe Drinking Water Act included a provision that required the EPA to "consider" the health of pregnant women, infants, and children in prioritizing chemicals for regulation and in setting standards. While this was a step forward, the EPA is required, nonetheless, to perform a cost-benefit analysis, the result of which can override the obligation to "consider" vulnerable populations in testing.[3] Although it seems obvious that the EPA should be setting a protective standard with the most vulnerable in mind, this research protocol is a reminder that standards set may not be shielding everyone from risk.[4]

The potential regulation of perchlorate even provides a window into America's party politics. Although there is a belief that the two parties have opposite worldviews on the environment and, therefore likely also, on drinking water, a close look at the record suggests otherwise. The differences may be one more of degree than absolutes.

In its decision making, the EPA's lack of urgency with perchlorate and with other drinking water contaminants has been a bipartisan policy failure for at least twenty-five years. While Democrats generally express more support for environmental safeguards, progress in speeding up decisions in drinking water regulation has been stymied through both Democratic and Republican administrations, and regardless of the party in control of Congress. Rhetorical and emotional support aside, only votes on bills can change funding and policies.

The EPA's on-again, off-again approach to regulating perchlorate is a primer in what has become of the goal of achieving safe drinking water since passage of the 1996 Amendments to the Safe Drinking Water Act. That long and inconclusive inquiry questioning whether to regulate perchlorate and at what level of concentration is but one example, even if, perhaps, the worst.

That case study follows.

Perchlorate Gets in Our Drinking Water

Perchlorate was first manufactured in Sweden in 1890. The laboratory creation is a far more concentrated version of the naturally occurring kind found mostly in Chile.[5] In its natural form, it has been used as fertilizer, and has been exported to farms around the world.[6] Production of the synthetic variety began in the U.S. in 1910, and due to the special properties of the synthetic version, it was employed, at least initially, only for fireworks and railroad signal flares.[7]

Perchlorate causes fuels to burn faster, hotter, and with more explosive power than they would if they were only drawing on available oxygen.[8] The chemical also mixes well with rubbery "binders" that can be molded to enhance consistency in manufacturing. Because of its oxygen-enhancing performance and its functionality in manufacturing, in the late 1940s, perchlorate was discovered to be ideal for a range of military functions. Before long, more than two hundred military applications using perchlorate were being manufactured for the U.S. armed forces and for export around the world. Some of these products include familiar items such as hand grenades, ejection seats for pilots, and rockets.[9]

Aside from its military uses, with the start of the U.S.-U.S.S.R. space race in the late 1950s, NASA also became a major customer of America's perchlorate manufacturers. To launch many of the rockets needed for the space program, NASA's engineers designed perchlorate-based, solid-fuel booster vehicles to get those American rockets off the ground faster and safer.[10]

Although about 90 percent of domestic perchlorate production is purchased by some department or agency of the U.S. government, the chemical is also used in many nonmilitary settings like mining, construction, fireworks, and academic earthquake research. In civilian life, perchlorate is most commonly used in highway safety flares and for fast opening of automotive air bags.[11] It's even utilized by criminal enterprises in the illegal production of methamphetamine.[12]

For a time, perchlorate had a medical application, as well. In 1952, researchers found perchlorate to be a valuable treatment for the overproduction of thyroid hormone, a disorder known as hyperthyroidism. When hyperthyroid patients were given doses of perchlorate dissolved in water, symptoms of the condition—like rapid heartbeat, sleeplessness, weight loss, and the development and growth of a goiter on the patient's neck—would often be reversed.[13] Today, perchlorate is no longer used in the U.S. for pharmaceutical purposes, but it had been a widely used drug for hyperthyroidism for about thirty years, finally giving way to other treatments.[14]

Until the late 1990s when precautionary steps began to be taken, wherever perchlorate was manufactured or used, its production or use was likely to pollute the groundwater. Nearly four hundred military sites around the country have been identified as having compromised groundwater from training exercises with weapons containing perchlorate, and from the disposal of those weapons after use or when they became obsolete.[15] At civilian facilities, such as where perchlorate was manufactured or where rockets or weapons were assembled under contract for NASA or the Pentagon, groundwater also often became contaminated, sometimes densely so.

Because perchlorate easily forms explosive mixtures, manufacturers of it used a lot of water to avoid any possibility of sparks inadvertently starting a fire during manufacturing. The water used for safety purposes, and all water utilized during production, would become contaminated with residues from contact with perchlorate.[16] To get rid of that tainted water, manufacturers employed a then-conventional, federal-government-approved form of wastewater treatment that might very well have been called the "Out of Sight, Out of Mind" system.

For example, at two of the largest perchlorate contract manufacturers, both located a short distance from Las Vegas in Henderson, Nevada, unlined evaporation ponds were built adjacent to factories to receive the water. Before the practice came to an end there in 1999, more than 18 billion gallons of contaminated water—bearing 21.5 million pounds of perchlorate residue—was discharged.[17] The water would either percolate into the sand or, as the name of the technique suggests, evaporate. Unknown to the designers of this inexpensive and seemingly effective wastewater treatment system, the perchlorate that was mixed with the wastewater didn't actually disappear.

Unlike the water with which it was mixed, none of the perchlorate residue evaporated. Because of the chemical structure of perchlorate, it dissolves easily in water and drains rapidly into the soil. In this way, without awareness of the environmental and public health consequences, millions of pounds of dissolved perchlorate entered into the ground—and from there into the groundwater. As the groundwater traveled, the perchlorate moved with it, creating, over time, an ever-greater circumference of contamination.

Very Small Amounts with the Potential to Cause Very Great Harm

No one seemed to give the Nevada practice of percolating perchlorate into the sand—or disposal of perchlorate anywhere—much thought until a technological innovation changed the way contaminants in water could be detected. In 1997, recently invented, highly sensitive measuring tools became able to detect even very small quantities of impurities.[18] As the devices grew more precise, scientists began detecting ever-lower volumes of contaminants, from parts per million to parts per billion. In more recent years, these tools could determine the presence of contaminants in water in parts per trillion. Some analytical chemists have begun doing work identifying pollutants in the parts per quadrillion, with the widespread use of measurements at that level within reach.[19]

To speak of tiny quantities of pollutants in our drinking water doesn't necessarily mean that they are harmless. Sometimes advocates of looser drinking water standards will say that a part-per-billion standard is akin to a sports stadium filled with golf balls, all of which but one is white. Or they will say that a parts-per-trillion standard is like an Olympic swimming pool in which the toxic material present equals the volume of one drop of water or a grain of salt. The use of these visual props is sometimes just for context, but it is often an intellectual sleight of hand, implying that such a small amount of contamination couldn't logically pose a threat to society. The examples imply that only a germaphobe or someone suffering from a compulsive disorder illness would seriously suggest that there is a need to rethink the approach to the safety of drinking water. But that doesn't match what we now know.

It may be true that some chemicals have no effect on (most of) us, or that they only affect us at certain points in our lives (such as in the womb, or as a newborn), or only harm us at high volumes. But it is also the case that very small amounts of a chemical consumed by the wrong person can create very bad health outcomes.

One example of this, even if not likely to be delivered via drinking water, has been tragically demonstrated in the ongoing opioid crisis. Unimaginably small amounts of fentanyl—the leading synthetic opioid—can kill quickly, with 1/14,000th of an ounce (0.0000705 of an ounce, or about half the weight of a grain of sand) of fentanyl recognized as a lethal dose for an adult of normal weight. Smaller, nonfatal amounts can bring on suppressed breathing and a drop in blood pressure in adults.[20] A child can have a variety of terrible outcomes, including death, with even less of the drug.[21]

Another example of a toxic element that is waterborne and can cause harm or kill at an even lower concentration than fentanyl is dioxin, a regulated drinking water contaminant. Dioxin may be best known as an element found at ultra-low levels in Agent Orange, used as a defoliant during the Vietnam War. It was later found to be the likely cause of leukemia in some of those who came into contact with it, and of birth defects in the children of some of those returning American soldiers. After ingestion of 1/30,000th of the weight of a single grain of salt, the sperm production of a 220-pound adult male can be disrupted by dioxin. It has also been shown to be fatal to a range of animals, again even at very low concentrations.[22]

Although a fatal single dose of perchlorate is essentially impossible, consumption of it, even in far smaller quantities than the example given with fentanyl or dioxin, has a predictable effect on our bodies. It blocks iodide—a form of iodine, and what is found in iodized salt, eggs, and seafood—from getting into the thyroid gland. If this occurs for a sustained period as short as a few weeks, it can lead to a shortfall in production of thyroid hormones, or a condition called hypothyroidism—the opposite, in a sense, of *hyper*thyroidism, in which too much of the thyroid hormone is produced. For most adults, the health implications of *hypo*thyroidism are relatively minor and easily reversed by changing diet or taking iodine supplements. But for newborns and for young children, and especially for fetuses through the first sixteen weeks of pregnancy, this endocrine system disruption and the suppression of iodide uptake—which can be caused by exposure to perchlorate at a small number of golf-balls-in-an-arena quantity—can be devastating. The harm done is irreversible.[23]

Unrelated to perchlorate, as much as 30 percent of pregnant women may have low iodide levels, mostly due to inadequate diet. When one of them drinks water with a sufficient dose of perchlorate in it during the first six weeks of pregnancy, it further suppresses her iodide levels, compounding the effects of the ingested perchlorate. Because of the short-fall of thyroid hormone caused by this iodide suppression, the unborn baby is exposed to the risk of birth defects, such as deficits in brain development. Although believed to be rare, the baby could be born with a variety of terrible outcomes, including the possibility of deafness or severe intellectual disability, which would be diagnosed soon after birth. It is also possible that the child won't have such grievous effects, but will have a lowered IQ or develop behavioral issues, which for any given individual can never be definitively traced back to a hormonal deficiency. The exposure causing the birth defects or other problems can come about directly from the mother to the fetus, or in infancy through drinking water or contaminated baby formula. Perchlorate can also be transferred via breast milk, making it possible for the newborn to be exposed while nursing, with the risk rising if the mother has ingested a high dosage of perchlorate.[24]

As is true of many diseases or hormonal disruptions caused by chemicals we ingest, no one can say for certain that a particular dose of perchlorate ingested by a pregnant woman or her new baby will result in a particular outcome. What long-term population studies make clear, though, is that in groups where pregnant and nursing mothers have higher levels of perchlorate in their urine, their children, as a group, have lower IQs and a variety of birth defects less likely to be found in similar groups where the women had low perchlorate levels.[25] Whether or not a golf-ball-in-an-arena amount is the tipping point for harm, it seems wise to have a protective standard that errs on the side of caution as even a very small disruption in the production of thyroid hormone in fetuses or infants can produce a lifetime of cognitive deficit.[26]

Meanwhile, the other image used to describe ultra-low levels of contaminants—the grain-of-salt-in-the-pool—seems to imply that it is nearly impossible to bring the volume of contaminants down any lower than it is already. But that mischievous idea is also false. With more filtration at drinking water treatment facilities, already low levels can be significantly reduced. The number could be brought to zero. That isn't a matter of technical know-how since the technology to achieve this already exists, but only a question of cost—a cost that some U.S. cities have already decided is worthwhile.[27] Or America could bring levels of new potentially hazardous contaminants down to zero by adopting the European toxic chemical control standard.

In Europe, generally speaking and not specific to any single chemical, the burden is supposed to be on the chemical company to prove that the chemical is harmless before it can be introduced, even if, in practice, implementation and enforcement of this approach has been irregular.[28] By contrast, in the U.S., all chemicals are welcomed into commerce unless and until they are proven to be harmful.[29] It is admittedly a hard balancing act as we do, after all, get great benefits from many chemicals, including perchlorate. But the American system has led more than a few critics to conclude that even toxic chemicals are considered "innocent until proven guilty" due to the permissive approach of putting commercial interests over that of public health concerns.[30]

"The Sins of the Fathers Came Home to Roost"

In February 1997, using recently invented, ultra-sophisticated equipment for detecting contaminants in water, a scientist with the California State Water Resources Board took a random sample of Colorado River water soon after it passed into his state.[31] He got a reading that showed the presence of perchlorate in the river. It wasn't a result he had expected.

The scientist had taken the sample as a control to be measured against a suspected contaminated site in southern California where solid-fuel rocket engines had been assembled for many years. His expectation was that the Colorado River perchlorate contamination level would be zero or so low as to be undetectable, even with his new, smart measuring tool. But getting a positive reading for perchlorate from the Colorado River was a surprise for another reason. Given the large volume of water in the river, the scientist assumed that the presence of any contaminant would be so diluted that, even using this new sensitive test, it wouldn't show a trace. The positive reading suggested that there must be a very dense source of perchlorate contamination upstream.[32]

Around that same time, water scientists in southern Nevada using similar screening tools took a reading of their own. They were looking for perchlorate in Lake Mead, and found high levels of contamination. Soon, the California and Nevada groups were working together, and they tracked perchlorate in reverse, from southern California up the Colorado River to Lake Mead and—no surprise—to the unlined evaporation ponds adjacent to the perchlorate factories there.

It quickly became clear that the perchlorate from the manufacturing process hadn't disappeared along with the water it had contaminated. Further, it seemed likely that the perchlorate was durable, with little or any of the chemical seeming to have broken down along the way. The intensity of the pollution was worse than anyone imagined possible. Utilizing test drillings into the soil, the water engineers soon figured out that, from its starting point in the unlined evaporation ponds in Henderson, Nevada, where the perchlorate had been manufactured, the chemical had traveled along with the groundwater, going east and slightly south to Lake Mead.[33]

Straddling Arizona and Nevada, the man-made Lake Mead was built in tandem with the Hoover Dam in the 1930s along the route of the

Colorado River.[34] Since its opening, it has been one of the most important water thoroughfares in the U.S., with a large role in the enormous growth of the population and economy of the Southwest.[35] By capacity, Lake Mead is the largest reservoir in the U.S., and it serves as a transit point for water to be used in farms and homes in southwestern Arizona, the southern (and most populous) parts of Nevada and California, and then into Mexico.

The lower Colorado River—as it is called from the spot it leaves Lake Mead until it reaches its endpoint—was the route of distribution for water, and unintentionally, for perchlorate, into a vast area in which much of America's high-quality produce is grown. It is also where about 25 million people live, including millions in southern California who get some of their drinking water from the lower Colorado River. In addition, Lake Mead provides 90 percent of the water consumed in Las Vegas and, ironically, all of the water used in Henderson, from where the contamination originated.[36]

"The sins of the fathers came home to roost," says Pat Mulroy, the longtime head of the Southern Nevada Water Authority. "Once we had the tools for figuring out what's in our water, we started finding contaminants that we'd never have had reason to know were there. But they were. Before that, we didn't know what we didn't know." And in the years since the discovery, with a long drought reducing the volume of Lake Mead, the perchlorate in the lake doesn't diminish because, "unlike the water, it doesn't evaporate," she says. But as the water level in Lake Mead drops due to drought, the density of perchlorate in the water there grows.

Beyond drinking water, researchers also found perchlorate in edible crops in California. "These fruits and vegetables are like a sponge," Mulroy says. "They absorb whatever is in the water you use to irrigate them with."[37] Tests have found perchlorate residues in broccoli, spinach, lettuce, tomatoes, and cucumbers, among other field crops irrigated with contaminated water.[38] As California's produce has a global market, presumably some of these fruits and vegetables were eaten far from where they were grown, yet further expanding the circle of contamination.

Mulroy is among the smartest and most experienced water practitioners in the U.S., and she is a fierce advocate for safe and abundant water. In 1999, just two years after the perchlorate was discovered in Lake Mead, she led a process in which Kerr-McGee, the larger of the Henderson perchlorate manufacturers, paid $1.1 billion into a trust fund to end further litigation. The fund has been used since then to remove and block as much perchlorate as possible from getting into the lake.

While the contamination persists to the present day, ongoing efforts underwritten by the trust fund have reduced the amount of perchlorate that flowed out of Lake Mead and back into the lower Colorado River. But relatively happy endings to stories of dense contamination are rare. Not every community facing contaminated water—whether perchlorate or some other toxic pollutant—has a Pat Mulroy, a deep pocket like Kerr-McGee, or a billion-dollar endowment to fund the effort to get rid of a persistent contaminant in the local water.

Yet, even as good as Mulroy is, and even with the most modern scientific and engineering techniques the settlement can buy, there are limits. "It is impossible to get rid of all of the perchlorate," she says. "It is impossible to get Lake Mead to zero. But what we can do is to bring the level down much lower than it was to where it is safe."[39]

Getting to agreement on how much perchlorate is safe in Nevada, California, and around the U.S. has proven to be harder, and taken longer, than anyone concerned about quality drinking water might have imagined possible.

The Pentagon's Assault on the EPA

Deciding the safe level for perchlorate, or any contaminant, in drinking water may sound like a task for an independent, conflicts-free, blue-ribbon scientific commission. Ideally, the panel would meet, review the current research, and set a standard. They might even offer revisions every few years as more scientific information became known. But our American system doesn't turn over decisions like these to impartial, highly qualified experts. Instead, we look to politicians and their appointees to make these important choices. Doctors and researchers may be called upon to provide advice to administrators and elected officials, some of whom may have relevant technical skills, but the decision to regulate or not—and at what level—is a political one.

The 1996 Amendments to the Safe Drinking Water Act created a high bar to regulating any contaminant. Aside from the cost-benefit analysis the EPA would be obliged to do, there were three separate decisions that the law required of the EPA. First, the chemical compound has to be shown to have an adverse effect on human health. Second, the contaminant must be frequently found in drinking water. And third, once both of those conditions are proven, the EPA must be able to demonstrate that by regulating the substance, there will be a "meaningful" opportunity to reduce the threat to public health.[40]

All three of these decisions are subjective. Congress offered no threshold for taking action or standard to use in making these judgments. As a result, the decision to regulate can, at least theoretically, cut either way. Looking at the same evidence, different EPA chiefs could legitimately come to opposite conclusions on whether to regulate or not. How bad must the effect be on public health? How frequently must the contaminant be found in drinking water? How many deaths, birth defects, instances of infertility, or other medical problems are needed to be "meaningful"? The law doesn't say.

Because of this lack of clarity, the decision about regulating perchlorate has bounced around for more than twenty years. At times, it looked like regulation was imminent, and at other times, it seemed there wasn't a chance it would ever occur. While there are significant economic consequences to regulation, there are also health risks incurred by the failure to regulate.

Deciding whether to regulate is only the first of two important decisions. As discussed briefly earlier, the other decision concerns the acceptable or "safe" level of contamination in drinking water. Since the EPA has almost never ruled that any contaminant's regulated level should be zero, the argument that follows whether a certain chemical compound should be regulated depends on what level of human intake of the contaminant is safe—and how costly "feasible" treatment technology is that can remove the contaminant from the water.

On both of these decisions, there are often two main opponents to regulation and to the setting of the "safe" contaminant threshold at a low concentration. Not surprisingly, the source of the contamination—the manufacturer, distributor, or industrial user—is one. The other group of opponents are the public water utilities, municipalities, and state governments. Such opposition by each is ordinarily motivated by cost, even if from different perspectives.

For the water utility, regulation of a contaminant means that the utility is obligated to test the water for the presence of that contaminant. If found, the level of toxicity has to be lowered by the water utility to the legal threshold before water can be distributed. Both the monitoring and the contaminant reduction may require new equipment or technology, adding unwanted expenses to the utility's budget.

The polluter looks at regulation and standard setting in a different way. Once the EPA issues a maximum safe level of a contaminant for drinking water, that threshold generally becomes the target level for cleanup at industrial waste sites.[41] If a chemical made, distributed, or used by a company is later regulated with a drinking water standard, the company can be compelled to pay to clean its polluting chemical at the site down to that maximum safe level set by the EPA's drinking water regulation. As a result, companies can face high cleanup charges of the environment going beyond water if the EPA sets a strict standard for a chemical manufactured, used, or disposed of by them.

With significant financial stakes tied to the decision, as long as the EPA doesn't put a particular chemical on its regulated contaminants list, the makers of the tens of thousands of chemicals used in daily life in the

U.S. are often free to do as they please, at least as regards protecting drinking water. Likewise, prior to that EPA determination, water utilities generally have no obligation to begin the monitoring or treatment referenced just above.[42] Each for its own reasons has significant motivation to delay or deny regulation.

Among chemicals found in drinking water, perchlorate is an unusual case. Unlike most other makers of waterborne contaminants, the perchlorate manufacturers have powerful partners who also have a reason to oppose regulation of perchlorate. The U.S. military, NASA, and the Department of Energy are the largest customers for perchlorate, and have been for several decades. No less than the perchlorate manufacturers, these three influential, well-funded parts of the federal government also benefit by any delay in perchlorate regulation.

One estimate has it that if perchlorate were to be regulated down to one part per billion—a possible science-based conclusion—it would require the Pentagon to spend $40 billion just to clean the contamination in the river bed of the lower Colorado River to that level.[43] This is money that would need to come out of other current and future spending by the Defense Department, resulting in less being available for the military's core mission. Further, while the Pentagon has taken steps to reduce perchlorate contamination at many of the nearly four hundred military and related government sites in the U.S. where it has been found, expenses for cleanup of the soil at these locations and elsewhere could mushroom if perchlorate were to be regulated at a lower level.[44]

While some presidents have treated the EPA as if it has cabinet-level status in the executive branch of the federal government, it doesn't have the power to act independently in the way other cabinet departments, such as the Department of Justice, do. The head of the EPA is appointed by the president, and all major decisions are presented to the president or the White House staff before they are made public.[45] Short of either an emergency or an inflamed public, presidents and their budget officials are generally reluctant to incur multi-billion-dollar liabilities by any part of their government.[46] As with a water utility or an industrial polluter, since significant (and expensive) ongoing pollution-control responsibilities would only start for a U.S. government department or agency after the EPA has regulated a contaminant and has set a maximum contaminant level, the government has no less incentive than the utility or polluting company to have the regulation of the contaminant rejected or delayed.

Benefiting the economic interests of water utilities and industrial or governmental polluters, the changes wrought by the 1996 Amendments to the Safe Drinking Water Act nearly guarantee that potentially harmful chemicals will not be regulated. In the decades since the passage of the 1996 Amendments, more than two hundred chemical compounds have been proposed for EPA review. Of these, including perchlorate, the EPA has selected only twenty-six for investigation, and of that small group of twenty-six, only perchlorate and one other have been chosen for possible regulation.[47] Neither has yet been regulated.

Will the regulation of perchlorate ever happen? Should it?

The Long Road to No Decision

Since 1992, the government, industry, and others have spent millions of dollars on more than one hundred research projects studying perchlorate and its effect on human health.[48] These tests continue even though it is settled science that, at sufficient doses, perchlorate suppresses the production of the thyroid hormone that blocks iodide absorption. It is also beyond dispute that, as a group, fetuses and newborns with reduced iodide levels have lower IQs and more developmental ills than those with normal thyroid hormone and iodide levels.[49]

The one test that would be of most value—on pregnant women and on newborn babies—is a test that can't be done because of the monstrous immorality it would present. No scientist so inclined to risk inflicting lifelong disability on a human subject could ever get permission to do such research. To mimic that un-doable experiment, researchers have performed toxicological studies using animals with physiological responses known to be similar to humans.

In 2002, scientists who had given rat fetuses and rat newborns infinitesimal doses of perchlorate via drinking water found that the rats had a wide range of developmental gaps and physical deformities.[50] The EPA believed the study was analogous to what would be the human response and, therefore, alarming for public health. Soon thereafter, the EPA set an advisory—that is, a nonbinding—threshold of one part per billion for perchlorate.[51]

If until then the pace of the federal investigation of perchlorate had been bureaucratic and glacial, the one-part-per-billion 2002 EPA advisory prompted an uncommonly rapid response by the U.S. government. A federal interagency group was convened consisting of representatives of the Defense Department, NASA, the Energy Department, and the White House Office of Management and Budget (OMB), along with the EPA and others, to discuss the economic implications of this low-threshold health advisory. As later revealed in documents discovered in litigation, at the meeting the Defense Department and OMB attempted to stop EPA action on perchlorate.[52] As a means of doing so, the federal interagency group recommended that yet another study be done, this one under the auspices of the U.S. National Research Council (NRC), which is a part of the National Academies of Sciences.

Although it is a prestigious organization, the NRC perchlorate study was controversial even before the committee issued its conclusions. Several key members of the research team had long-standing business ties to the Pentagon, NASA, or one of the perchlorate manufacturers, a potential conflict that safe drinking water advocates believed disqualified them, especially as those conflicts had not been disclosed.[53] Whether those conflicts were actually relevant or not, the NRC report, issued in January 2005, relied upon an industry-funded study of thirty-seven adults exposed to perchlorate and rejected the protective one-part-per-billion standard set by the EPA in 2002 based upon the earlier animal research.

The NRC report concluded that the presence of perchlorate in drinking water was safe up to 24.5 parts per billion, a permissible volume nearly twenty-five times greater than what the EPA had proposed following the 2002 research report. In January 2006, using the NRC study as its justification, the EPA reversed its prior advisory level for perchlorate and issued a new advisory opinion, adopting the far more relaxed 24.5-parts-per-billion standard recommended by the NRC.

Two months after the EPA set the higher standard, in March 2006 the EPA's Children's Health Protection Advisory Committee—an independent body of medical and scientific professionals—sent a letter to the head of the EPA raising the failure of the NRC study to adequately take into account the health risk to fetuses, newborns, and young children. The risk to fetuses aside, the letter made the observation that since perchlorate passes through the body, and is also found in breast milk, nursing babies might be exposed to yet higher levels of perchlorate than only from drinking water.[54]

Likewise, the EPA advisory committee's letter said that giving babies formula might also be risky. Since it was impossible to be sure if reconstituted formula had perchlorate mixed in from the tap water used, there was no clarity on the dosage babies were getting. And because there was no ongoing monitoring of perchlorate levels by water utilities and effort by them to remove perchlorate when found, it was a possibility that even pre-mixed formula could come from baby food and baby formula factories that had perchlorate-contaminated water. To protect the health of these newborns and babies, the letter concluded, prudence demanded that a highly restrictive standard be set.[55]

The EPA fell back into a period of study and review. In January 2007, the agency announced that it had all of the data it needed to make a decision, and in the last months of the second term of George W. Bush, in October 2008, the EPA announced it would not be regulating perchlorate after all.[56] The EPA statement said that—notwithstanding perchlorate being found in drinking water at 153 utilities in 28 states—contamination was not widespread enough to merit national regulation and that, in any event, it did not believe regulating perchlorate would have a meaningful effect on health.[57]

Twenty Years, and Counting

Within a month of the administration of Barack Obama coming into office in January 2009, the EPA announced that it was taking a fresh look at the possibility of regulating perchlorate. After the roller coaster of the Bush years in which perchlorate went from being given an advisory threshold of one part per billion to having a new proposed standard of 24.5 parts per billion, and then, in the administration's closing days in 2008, to having perchlorate taken off the list of potential regulated contaminants altogether, the Obama EPA announcement could be seen as the last step before perchlorate would finally be monitored and controlled.

Those eager to have perchlorate—or any contaminant—regulated were also likely elated when the EPA announced in February 2011 that it had determined perchlorate posed a threat to the health of as many as 16 million Americans and that regulation of it could meaningfully reduce that risk.[58] In what was as close to a sure thing in the world of drinking water, it looked like perchlorate would finally be a regulated contaminant, even if the maximum contaminant level—one part per billion or 24.5 parts per billion, or something in between—was still unknown. The 2011 announcement committing to setting of a standard, made in the first Obama term, was referring to an event that wouldn't occur before the end of what would be a second Obama term, assuming that he won reelection.

After that February 2011 EPA declaration that perchlorate would be regulated, the next steps were clear. The Safe Drinking Water Act requires the setting of a preliminary maximum contaminant level within two years of the initial determination, and a final contaminant threshold by no later than eighteen months after that.[59] In other words, by August 2014, it should have all been completed.

But it wasn't finished then, or at all during the Obama years.

The EPA announcements in 2009 and 2011 may both have been sincere. Delay could have been caused because the EPA was understaffed, or lacking in adequate funds, or distracted by other environmental threats, or the science around perchlorate regulation may have proven more daunting than they first imagined. But based on what was soon revealed in court about the Pentagon and NASA still being opposed to perchlorate regulation, it isn't impossible to imagine that internal maneuvering in the Obama White House played a part here, too.

If what the law required had been followed, perchlorate would have already been added to the list of regulated contaminants by the end of Obama's second term, and no future administration could have easily reversed that. Yet by February 2016, nearly two years after the drinking water statute demanded it all be completed, it still wasn't. This led the Natural Resources Defense Council (NRDC), an environmental public interest organization, to sue the EPA to compel the agency to set a perchlorate standard.

During court proceedings, the attorney for the U.S. government volunteered that resolution of regulation of perchlorate was being delayed because of "different views" by NASA and the Defense Department, with the implication that they were a key reason for the delay.[60] But with no legal defense available, the government attorney agreed to a request by the NRDC that the judge issue an order compelling the EPA to set a final standard by December 2019.[61]

Whether perchlorate will be regulated by that newest date is unknowable at the time of this writing. But with more than twenty years of review, a further delay should not surprise those who have followed this story. With the administration of Donald Trump making relief from environmental regulations a key part of its economic policy, it is possible that perchlorate will, again, be taken off the list of contaminants to regulate, forcing a new start to the process by some future administration, if ever. Or a Trump EPA could set a standard so high—at, say, 80 parts per billion, or higher—that it would have no real-world impact on water treatment and only a modest budgetary impact on the Pentagon or NASA for cleaning up contaminated sites.

Should December 2019 come and go without regulation of perchlorate, one alternative could be for states to pick up where the federal government has failed to lead. Already California and Massachusetts have set mandatory perchlorate drinking water limits within their states of six and two parts per billion, respectively, and both have set even more ambitious aspirational goals.[62]

In addition, eighteen other states have some form of oversight of perchlorate, whether mandatory notice above a stated level or advisory guidance.[63] If the EPA fails to follow through, other states will likely join the list of those concerned about perchlorate. Ironically, a return to a pre-Safe Drinking Water Act world in which states are primarily responsible for water safety guidelines may protect the largest number of people, at least as regards perchlorate.

"It may be easier for states to regulate a contaminant than for the EPA to do so," says Dr. Melanie Marty, a veteran senior official in California's state environmental agency and a toxicology expert who has long followed the starts and stops in perchlorate regulation. "The EPA gets a ton more political pressure than does any state environmental agency. There are more stakeholders looking at what they are doing than in any state, and they get more comments. The staff there is very thorough and they go through each one, and that causes delays." Even so, the real difference, Dr. Marty says, is the political pressure on the EPA from the perchlorate industry and from federal departments like the Pentagon that could be liable for expensive cleanups.[64]

Yet counting on states to take on regulation of drinking water contaminants may also be unlikely. With state and local governments facing current budget challenges—and with vocal, well-organized constituencies for education, welfare, health care, police, and transportation, among other areas, making claims on scarce taxpayer dollars— some states and cities aren't eager to add to their financial burdens to address a concern like perchlorate that is neither in the news nor which has the attention of an aggrieved and dedicated bloc of voters. State and local government officials would prefer to not take on or add water fees to fund advanced water treatment, even at amounts of less than a dollar a week per person.

But there may be another solution, and that is to stop permitting the perfect to be the enemy of the good. As Dr. Melanie Marty, the California toxicologist, suggests, maybe we would do better to change our approach. "While we are waiting for some perfect study that tells us what to do," she says, "we are leaving populations exposed to contaminants."

What can be safely said is that, by now, after more than twenty years of investigation into perchlorate, the EPA should have made a decision. During those twenty years—through Democratic and Republican presidencies and through Democratic and Republican majorities in Congress, and despite the thousands of newly created chemicals and the tens of thousands that predate this period—not one chemical has been added to the EPA's regulated chemical contaminant list for drinking water. Perchlorate shouldn't be added simply to make a statement or for symbolic purposes, but neither should a process—for perchlorate or any chemical—be permitted to drag on for so long.

"If there are those who think the level has been set too low," Dr. Marty says speaking about perchlorate, but with advice that applies more generally, "let them continue to do scientific research. If we made a mistake, if the level got set too low, it can be set higher. But you need to set a standard, and if you are doing it, it's best to be overly health protective. If the science gets smarter, let's change it then."[65]

PART II

THE CHALLENGE

Four

PILLS IN THE WATER

"There is evidence that we are being exposed to lots of
pharmaceutical products at low levels—sub-therapeutic levels. . . .
We don't know who is drinking it or in what combinations
or amounts."
—Dr. Luke Iwanowicz

D R. LUKE IWANOWICZ, a research biologist with the U.S. Geological Survey (USGS), looks at human health from an unusual angle. Because it is often difficult to understand the long-term effects of chemical contaminants on humans, he examines fish that have been in contact with those same compounds and sees how—if at all—they are affected. To mix metaphors, he sees fish as the canary in the coal mine. They are a proxy, or sentinel, for potential coming threats. At a minimum, his tests reveal if fish are in danger; at most, he finds out if we are.

Not content to only look at fish, Iwanowicz looks at the ecosystem in which those fish live. And among the most significant contributors to contaminants getting into that ecosystem are the more than fourteen thousand wastewater treatment plants around the U.S. Unless connected to a septic system, what goes down the sink, shower, bath, dishwasher, washing machine, and toilet is transferred to one of these facilities. The plants do a very good job of neutralizing microorganisms in the sewage that can make us sick or foul our waterways, but they have failed to keep up with lifestyle changes from the time when most of them were designed and built.

One such major lifestyle change is the widespread use of pills and other medications.

The U.S. started the twentieth century with few common medications other than codeine, a remedy that had long been available for coughs and as an all-purpose anesthetic. Aspirin was invented in Germany in 1897 and introduced in the U.S. a few years later. Targeted painkillers were invented in the 1920s. But, overall, consumers were largely left to home remedies—and prayer—for a range of ailments and concerns. But it is a very different story today.

Each day, Americans swallow a mountain of pills. Nearly 60 percent of those who are eighteen years old and over take at least one prescription pill every day, and 16 percent take five or more.[1] One cholesterol-lowering medication is taken by 8 percent of all adults, and one in six Americans takes some form of psychiatric medicine, whether an antidepressant, an antianxiety, or an antipsychotic pill.[2] Antibiotics are prescribed nearly 270 million times each year—enough for five of every six Americans.[3]

The framework for all of this is vast. Aside from the drug companies, many of which are among the world's largest corporations, there are more than 52,000 prescription medicines approved by the Food and Drug Administration (FDA) that are available for sale, and more than 5,000 over-the-counter drugs on the market.[4] In the most recent year for which data is available, America's 300,000 pharmacists working in 61,000 pharmacies dispensed nearly 4.4 billion prescriptions.[5] Total annual U.S. spending on prescription medicines, which is projected to keep growing, is already nearly $330 billion, making it one of the largest consumer product categories.[6]

A pill-popping America isn't necessarily bad news, especially if done responsibly and under a doctor's guidance. People get to live longer and have a better quality of life. The problem, at least from the perspective of safe drinking water, is what happens to the nation's water supply after each of those pills is swallowed.

Because pharmaceutical products are inefficiently absorbed by the body, within a few hours, up to 90 percent of the pill is discharged as bodily waste. The drug companies understand how inefficient their products are and, to hit the intended target, nearly every pill has more drug in it than is needed.[7] All of that surplus ends up in the toilet or, when sweated out, in the shower drain or washing machine. Compounding the problem, many prescriptions either get changed or not finished, and many patients or caregivers flush the leftover pills down the toilet to dispose of them. Whether ingested or disposed of, soon thereafter the pharmaceutical residues from these pills travel to the local wastewater treatment plant.

Since the nation's wastewater treatment plants rarely use existing technology to remove the chemicals in those pills, the remains of the medicines are then discharged to nearby waterways. Over time, the wastewater from your home—and the contaminants in it—can travel great distances, but can also end up in your or someone else's tap water.

A March 2008 study that checked the drinking water of twenty-eight major metropolitan U.S. regions found pharmaceutical products in the drinking water of twenty-four of them, putting 41 million people at risk.[8] A second round of testing later that year in twenty-seven additional, but smaller, cities found drug residues in seventeen of them, adding five million more to those found to have pharmaceutical contaminants in their drinking water.[9] Beyond this total group of 46 million, there is an unknown number who live outside of one of those markets, but who are also possibly consuming someone else's prescription drug residues.

If a lake is your community's largest nearby body of water, your treated wastewater may be sent there with most of these pharmaceutical residues still present in some form. At another part of the lake, your community would likely draw its drinking water. Likewise, if your town or city discharges its treated wastewater into a river, everyone downriver of you is at risk of encountering those contaminants in their own drinking water, just as your drinking water is at risk from the untreated contaminants from places upriver of you. The farther down the river, the greater the risk. But nearly everyone is downriver of someone else's wastewater treatment plant and the remains of that community's pharmaceutical usage.

Estrogen and Its Doppelgängers

One pill in particular—a pill so iconic in American life that it is simply called "The Pill"—contributes, in the aggregate, to a significant amount of hormones in wastewater and, potentially, in drinking water. Since its introduction in 1960, birth control pills have, in one form or another, been a staple prescription drug. Today, nearly 27 percent of American women who are avoiding pregnancy take a birth control pill, a dose of synthetic estrogen that tricks a woman's body's endocrine system and suppresses ovulation. That one variety of pill, taken for twenty-one days out of every twenty-eight, adds over 10 million doses to America's wastewater every day.[10]

In addition to the women taking birth control pills, there are millions of other women beyond child-bearing age who take estrogen and other hormone supplements to help moderate the effects of menopause. Even after a series of cancer scares led to a nearly 60 percent drop in the use of estrogen replacement therapy, more than four million American women still take a daily regimen of hormonal supplements to mitigate menopausal conditions. At one point, though, in the early 2000s, more than 20 million women in the U.S. were taking hormones as birth control pills, as a means of regulating menstruation, or to moderate the effects of menopause. Currently, usage by those groups has been reduced to a still sizable total population of around 15 million regular users, but at whatever level of usage, all of these pills add to the total residue of estrogen hormones in the water.[11]

Since women aren't the only ones ingesting these chemicals, the volume of hormones that can be contaminating our water is far higher.[12] Livestock are fed estrogen or other similar hormones to promote growth and, in the case of dairy cows, they are often treated with hormones to boost milk production.[13] Similar to humans, within hours of these millions of animals ingesting these drugs, the hormones are eliminated.

In addition, cows and other female livestock naturally produce estrogen, and this is also excreted. Whether transported to a local waterway after some form of water treatment at a feedlot or eliminated as animal waste and absorbed by the soil to percolate into groundwater, the residues of all of this estrogen also contribute to the total.

Beyond estrogen from birth control pills and farm animals, there is another potentially massive source of estrogen that is likely getting into source water. Iwanowicz, the U.S. Geological Survey research biologist, explained how some benign lab creations are also adding to the threat of estrogen, or estrogen-like, exposure.

"There are many chemicals designed for specific, nonestrogenic biological functions," says Iwanowicz, "but by coincidence they, too, function like estrogens, usually 'weak estrogens.' This is generally the case because the geometry [of the newly designed chemical] is similar enough to estrogen that they share some biological function. These are chemical doppelgängers of sorts."[14]

Although these chemicals were engineered in labs for an entirely different purpose than to serve as or to mimic estrogen, "they have the capacity," Iwanowicz says, "to interfere with the normal functioning of the body, including reproductive and sexual health, as well as other possible consequences, like obesity, diabetes, and behavioral issues."[15]

These estrogenic compounds include many herbicides and pesticides as well as some plastic products, cosmetics, and industrial solvents, among others.[16] And although they are not as "bioactive as pure estrogen, they get into the water supply in great quantities," Iwanowicz said. Although weaker as an estrogen than a chemical designed as estrogen, such as the birth control pill, these estrogenic compounds may be of more concern than estrogen itself. Estrogen derived from pills and animal feed gets degraded "over weeks or months, and certainly within years," Iwanowicz said, "but because many [of these chemicals] are designed to withstand sunlight and a variety of weather conditions, they don't degrade as easily as does the estrogen in a birth control pill. Those estrogenic chemicals can be with us for a long time."[17]

While the effect on humans of all of this estrogen and estrogen-like compounds in surface water is still unknown, Iwanowicz and his fish biologist colleagues have seen what effect it seems to be having on fish. If those fish are harbingers of things to come for humans and other species—something that can only be known with more research—we would be wise to begin making use of technologies already in hand to reduce the estrogen that gets into our source water, and from there into our drinking water.

Fish and Their Grandparents

Despite its name, the lakes, rivers, ponds, and reservoirs that make up the U.S. National Wildlife Refuge System aren't all located in the wild or far from civilization. In the Northeast, some parts are pristine, while other elements of the so-called refuges are found near suburban communities. One is even close to a small airport. This diversity of locations—and varied conditions of remoteness and purity—served Iwanowicz's purposes in the design of research trying to investigate the presence of estrogen, and the effect, if any, on fish found at each of nineteen separate waterways.[18]

After confirming the presence of estrogen at most of the nineteen locations, Iwanowicz collected both largemouth and smallmouth bass from their refuge habitats for examination. Between 60 and 100 percent

of the male smallmouth bass caught and studied were found to have begun developing female characteristics, primarily the presence of eggs adjacent to the male sex organs. The phenomenon of an animal of a defined
sex developing sexual apparatus, or biomarkers, most commonly associated with the other sex is called intersexuality.[19]

There were differences in the abnormalities in the fish Iwanowicz
studied. Some, he speculates, were simply more susceptible to an adverse
reaction to the contaminants. But one pattern that held constant in all
river refuges that were surveyed was that intersex severity was found to
be higher at downriver locations. It would be there, presumably, that
greater concentrations of the endocrine-disrupting estrogen would be
found from streams feeding into those rivers and carrying estrogen (and
other contaminants) from points unknown. Generally, contamination
tends to get worse the farther one travels downriver, possibly with worse
health consequences experienced in downriver locales where more concentrated levels of contaminants are found.

In related fish research done by colleagues of Iwanowicz, estrogen in
the water is believed to have wreaked havoc with the hormonal systems
of those fish species under investigation. In one study, sex ratios skewed
female, and in other studies, impaired sperm density and lower sperm
quality were discovered among male fish.[20] Not surprisingly, widespread
reproductive failure was found. Reinforcing the greater hazard of being
a consumer of downstream water, in one of the fish studies, no intersex
fish were found upriver above where a municipal wastewater treatment
plant discharged its treated sewage. Downriver of the treatment plant,
though, about 20 percent of the fish population studied was found to be
intersex. In that same river, the male population downriver was half of
what it was upriver.[21]

Iwanowicz offers another possible explanation for the intersexuality
that he and the others have found in their studies. Perhaps the relevant
variable isn't the amount of current exposure to estrogen and other contaminants endured by the fish examined by these scientists. "In seeing
this disruption to the fish endocrine systems," Iwanowicz says, "we may

be witnessing a multigenerational effect. It could be that the parents or grandparents of the intersex fish were exposed to hormones or other contaminants and that those chemical compounds altered their genes. The intersexuality of their children or grandchildren could be a delayed, or epigenetic, result of that exposure."

Fish—or their parents and grandparents—may be uniquely sensitive to estrogen and other elements found in their water. But they might not be the only species undergoing estrogen-driven hormonal changes. Since the EPA doesn't require water utilities to test for the presence of estrogen, it would be valuable to know how much estrogen and estrogenic chemicals are getting into our drinking water. Likewise, for other pharmaceutical residues.

If scientific prudence keeps Iwanowicz from making a definitive statement linking specific risks for humans from waterborne contaminants, his experience with fish as sentinels seems to have, nonetheless, given him a sense of alarm. "There is evidence that we are being exposed to lots of pharmaceutical products at low levels—sub-therapeutic levels—but in a cocktail," he says, referring to a mixture of chemicals coming together. "As a result, predicting the outcome of this exposure is impossible. The concentration of these chemicals isn't measured [by the EPA] in drinking water and we don't know who is drinking it or in what combinations or amounts. It's like a black box with water going into a pipe and we don't know exactly what comes out of it. But we know that we need to learn a lot more, because throwing caution to the wind isn't a good strategy."[22]

The Solution to Pollution Isn't Dilution

The Great Lakes are, by far, the largest single source of freshwater in the U.S. Spanning nearly one thousand miles—from Minnesota in the west to New York in the east—eight states and Canada's Ontario province border the lakes. Representing more than a fifth of the world's surface freshwater, the five lakes taken together equal nearly 85 percent of all of the surface water in the continental U.S.[23] As of now, about 35 million people get their drinking water from the Great Lakes, but should it ever become necessary, and if the Great Lakes states would agree to share their bounty, the nearly limitless capacity of these inland freshwater seas could provide sustenance for many millions more.[24]

One of the arguments sometimes made against more comprehensive treatment of sewage is that the contaminants that survive the process are often received by large bodies of water. As such, the argument goes, the density of the contaminants is brought down to a level where they can no longer be harmful. Advocates of this approach are fond of using a cheerful, if simplistic, rhyme—"The solution to pollution is dilution"— to make their point.

If there has ever been a place to test this premise, it's unlikely a better venue could be found than the Great Lakes to do so. With their oceanic volume of water, surely, the advocates of the "solution-to-pollution" position would say, the discharges of the 1,448 Great Lakes region wastewater treatment plants—which produce 4.8 billion gallons of treated wastewater every day—and the drainage from over 126,000 farms of all sizes covering 55 million acres of agricultural land would be rendered unmeasurable and, even if measurable, then safe.[25]

But the opposite might also be true. If the contaminants that flow into the Great Lakes—whether after surviving processing at wastewater treatment plants or being the result of agricultural runoff—are both measurable and dangerous, it would be a signal that far smaller bodies of water are being contaminated, or certainly at risk of being so, unless and until the contaminants are neutralized.

Professor Diana Aga has come a long way from her remote village in the Philippines where she grew up without electricity or running water to being a world-renowned analytical chemist recognized for her work with a chaired professorship at the State University of New York at Buffalo.

She began her career looking at pesticide residues in Lake Superior but moved on to study an array of pharmaceutical products, growing ever more concerned about the risks they present individually and collectively.

She recently completed a fish research project in the Great Lakes. "Fish are highly relevant subjects for study," Aga says. "What happens often is that effects are seen first on birds or fish, and later on with more complex creatures."[26]

Her project had her looking generally for contaminants in ten fish species found in the Great Lakes. While several contaminants were found in the muscle of the fish—that is, the part that Americans are most likely to eat—those same contaminants were also found in the brains and organs. What jumped out at her and her fellow researchers was that antidepressants were found in the brains of at least some representatives from all ten species, and in more than half of all fish tested regardless of species. Multiple residues from well-known brand names like Prozac, Celexa, and Zoloft were present in some fish as well as many generic forms of antidepressants.

Asked to explain the significance of her study, Aga methodically ticks off key points. "First, unlike with some drugs that are both used by humans and animals," she says, "these antidepressants aren't coming from farms and farm animals. Second, it means that these residues are coming from wastewater treatment plants that drain into the Great Lakes. Third, it means that the wastewater treatment plants aren't preventing these pharmaceutical products from getting into surface water. And finally, this means that even in very large bodies of water, these products are getting into what is the source for drinking water, and at levels high enough to be measurable across all species studied."

The problem seems only to be growing. From 2000 to 2015, the use of antidepressants in the U.S. rose by 65 percent.[27] "We saw this significant change in usage levels happening in front of us," Aga says, "and we have done nothing to improve the removal of them at the wastewater treatment plants. Even if we don't know with certainty what the long-term effects here will be, it is reasonable to say that significant amounts of antidepressants and other pharmaceuticals are getting into surface water at ever greater concentrations and that it could be getting into drinking water. But since the EPA doesn't regulate the levels of pharmaceuticals in drinking water sources, we don't know to what extent our drinking water is being affected by these contaminants."

Aga isn't only concerned about antidepressants. She has worked in many other areas of analytical chemistry, where she has researched the presence of household products and a wide range of drugs in water. With years of experience, she steps out of her lab to share her worldview. "There are many chemical compounds that aren't regulated and which are called 'emerging contaminants,'" she says. "They have been 'emerging' for so long that we've all come to take them for granted. People ask me, 'Why are you focused on this? No one will die from drinking water that has them in it.'"

But Aga believes that death isn't the only consideration that should be of concern, as there may be other serious consequences. Even if not seen today, she says, these may just take a long time to reveal themselves or skip a generation.

"We are seeing ever greater instances of endocrine disruption in individuals," she says. "Our children could be affected by these compounds in our drinking water. Some girls are entering into puberty younger, and with unknown effects later in life. We suspect boys have lower sperm counts, but we don't know for sure.[28] Many children exposed to these 'emerging contaminants' could be suffering from lower IQs, learning disabilities, ADHD, even autism. All of these are consequences of interference, very possibly from contaminants in the water, with the body's self-regulating endocrine system."

In addition to the possible effects of contaminants on individuals, Aga is gravely concerned about ever-greater levels of antibiotic resistance that may also be coming from drinking water sources polluted with antibiotic residues. Harmful bacteria, also known as pathogens, adapt to antibiotics, and in recent years these pathogens have been developing defenses to antibiotics more quickly than the world's scientists and pharmaceutical companies can develop yet more powerful drugs. In a race against time, the bacteria, with their superior adaptability, seem to be beating the human beings, with our (supposedly) superior intellects.

"There is reason to believe that by the year 2050, the number one killer won't be cancer," Aga says, "but infections from bacterial pathogens, so-called superbugs, that can't be stopped with existing antibiotics. We've been in an era since the 1950s where pathogens could be easily eliminated with antibiotics in the form of a pill, a shot, or an IV drip. If those treatments go away, we will return to an era where people can die from simple infections, and the possibility of deadly epidemics returns."

When antibiotics are properly prescribed to treat an infection, some bacteria that are the intended targets are not neutralized. Those that survive then reproduce and their offspring can withstand another exposure to the same antibiotic. They also travel from one human to another. When an antibiotic fails to perform as intended, as is happening with greater frequency, doctors are obliged to use different and ever-stronger antibiotics to try to kill the smarter, more adaptable pathogens. Already, about 23,000 Americans die each year from antibiotic-resistant bacteria; at some point there will be no remaining antibiotics to which the bacteria haven't developed resistance.[29] This is the "post-antibiotic era" about which the World Health Organization has expressed alarm.[30]

A similar, if more dangerous, process occurs when drinking water contains sub-therapeutic levels of antibiotics. Bacterial pathogens that may be in the water supply or may be in our bodies at low levels, or even benign bacteria, get to experience the antibiotic at exceptionally low doses and begin to adapt to it. When the person gets an infection and is prescribed one of the relative handful of current antibiotics, the pathogens have already developed an immunity. They aren't neutralized, and the infection or fever can grow worse, possibly culminating in death. As such, even trace amounts of antibiotics in drinking water or our bodies can accelerate the process of antibiotic resistance.

"There is no question that we should be upgrading our nation's wastewater treatment plants and drinking water treatment facilities," Aga says. "When they were built, there were specific threats, and they addressed those threats. Now, there are new threats. We need to address those new threats, and we can with existing engineering technologies."

The Health Hazard from Your Local Health Facility

Hospitals, nursing homes, assisted living residences, and hospices all have something in common: Their patients and residents are likely to be nearly universal users of medicines. When the Clean Water Act was passed in 1972 and an effort was made to reduce the flow of pollutants into the nation's lakes and rivers, it would have made sense to have put hospitals into a category like factories or feedlots. Both factories and feedlots produce dense pollution and, following passage of the law, both were required to remediate their wastewater before discharging it. But at that time, there wasn't an awareness of the dangers to drinking water from pharmaceutical contaminants. As a result, it never came up in congressional hearings or committee meetings.[31]

In the nearly fifty years that have followed, federal water law continues to mostly give hospitals a free pass, allowing them and other health-related facilities to dispose of their wastewater not much differently than an ordinary homeowner connected to the municipal water grid. Regardless of size of facility or department function, hospitals flush their mix of high-powered pharmaceutical agents and antibacterial cleaning products down the drain or toilet—and into the municipal water supply.[32]

It isn't as if hospitals and other medical facilities aren't already forced to be mindful of the environmental consequences of their activities. Hospitals are required to segregate their solid medical waste. Items like used syringes, bloody bandages, lab-tested benign human tissue, and even tongue depressors are all required to be segregated and carted separately from the rest of the hospital's trash.[33] After removal from the hospital, a variety of state and local laws and regulations govern how to dispose of these potentially infectious or hazardous solid waste products. But there is no comparable requirement for hospital wastewater.[34]

With over 900,000 beds in more than 5,600 U.S. hospitals, each year nearly 21 million patients stay an average of between five and six days.[35] While in the hospital, a patient is likely to receive treatment with one or more high-potency medications. Cancer patients may receive chemotherapy, a treatment that utilizes drugs designed to kill human cells. Patients of all kinds may be sent for tests that include MRIs and CT scans, often requiring the patient to take radio-contrast media to make those tests easier to read. Contrast media can produce intense allergic reactions. If the patient is in the hospital for surgery, they are sure to receive some form of anesthesia, and patients of all kinds receive narcotics and other pain medication. Anesthetics and pain medication each have a targeted effect on the central nervous system. More than half of all U.S. hospital patients are given at least one antibiotic drug during their stay, with many of them receiving the most powerful form of antibiotic that now exists via an intravenous drip.[36] But regardless of the cause for the hospital admission, or the length of stay, and whether by pill, injection, or IV drip, hospitalized patients routinely receive some form of medication in one of seventeen categories of pharmaceutical compounds.[37]

Beyond the significant volume of medicines that hospitals administer to patients that inevitably find their way into the hospital wastewater, doctors and hospital staff routinely use antimicrobial products on their hands that are typically washed down hospital sinks. Operating rooms and hospital floors are regularly washed with strong, antimicrobial solutions. Many hospitals also have special laundries to be sure that the bacteria on patients' sheets don't survive the wash cycle.[38]

As a result of all of these dosing and sterility practices, hospitals produce a large volume of pharmaceutical and other toxic waste. While Americans outside of hospitals consume (and discharge) a far larger amount of medication than do those in hospitals, the wastewater leaving a hospital is certain to contain more dangerous chemicals and in a denser concentration than any comparable water sample from the same number of people elsewhere.[39]

Hospitals aren't the only community health venues producing highly concentrated wastewater filled with toxic matter. Over the past forty years, there has been a net decline of about two thousand U.S. hospitals.[40] The reasons are many, and, except for waves of consolidations made for business purposes, reflect mostly good news in medical care, like advances in less-intrusive surgery, the rise of effective medicines, and implantable medical devices. One additional reason for the decline in hospitals during these forty years is that—due to the rise of alternative care centers such as hospices—end-of-life patients no longer need to be in hospitals, places better suited to curing patients and not just managing the pain of their last days and weeks.

The first hospice in the U.S. was opened in 1974, two years after the passage of the Clean Water Act. As hospices demonstrated that they could fill an important need for patients and their families, their numbers grew. Today, there are nearly 4,400 hospices caring for about 1.2 million patients each year. The average stay is a bit over two months.[41]

As with hospitals, hospices are pharmaceutical-centric enterprises. On the National Hospice and Palliative Care Organization's list of "major responsibilities," the first item is management of "patient's pain," and the third item is providing "needed drugs."[42] Keeping patients pain-free often requires keeping them numbed or sedated by round-the-clock administration of narcotics and other medicines. As with hospitals, hospices have no obligation to filter their wastewater, creating a residue rich in narcotics and sedatives, along with antibiotics and other medicines.

Nursing homes and assisted living facilities are also found in every American community of any significant-sized population. And while neither of those necessarily prescribes drugs with the same intensity as do hospitals and hospices, both, by definition, are home to older people. About half of Americans aged seventy-five and older take statins to reduce cholesterol, 40 percent take blood pressure medication, and 16 percent take pain medication on a daily basis.[43] In 2015, the EPA estimated that America's nursing homes throw away about 740 tons of medication each year, with at least four times as much consumed by the patients themselves at those facilities.[44]

Where once it seemed onerous to demand that factory owners clean their water before discharging it, every manufacturing plant has long been required to have a water remediation plan. With a witches' brew of compounds coming from health care facilities, the public's health and safety could be put less at risk, and source water less prone to pharmaceutical contamination, if hospitals, hospices, nursing homes, and assisted living facilities were required to detoxify their wastewater—or the wastewater of key departments—before flushing it down the communal drain.

Landfills and Septic Systems: Conduits for Contamination

Not every pill that is prescribed ends up being swallowed. Each year, an estimated 200 million pounds of medication go unused, creating the problem of how to best dispose of it.[45] For sure, unused prescriptions can't be permitted to get into the hands of those who would make use of drugs without a doctor's guidance. But the unused medicines can also become a threat to drinking water quality.

A small amount of unused drugs gets returned to pharmacies that have "Take Back" projects, programs to arrange for the safe disposal of prescription medicines. Once a critical volume of the returned drugs is amassed, the pharmacy arranges for the pills to be incinerated, usually to then have the ashes placed in a landfill. But these programs are often not as effective as may be hoped. One federal study concluded that states often fail to properly destroy the prescription medicines collected.[46]

"Take Back" programs aside, a far larger amount of unused medicines is flushed down the toilet. This results in those drugs going to the municipal wastewater treatment plant or septic tank similar to what would happen to those drugs when taken and then excreted by the patient. But without advanced water treatment at the wastewater facility, most or all of the chemical compounds in the pills can survive. Much of those surviving pharmaceutical residues end up in lakes and rivers as part of the discharge from the treatment plant.

More even than incineration or disposal down the toilet, likely the largest amount of unused medicine is thrown out with the trash. Those pills soon end up in a landfill. Some conscientious consumers pulverize the pills and mix them with soil or coffee grounds to make sure that no one else can use the unprescribed medicines, but regardless of whether or not they are adulterated, the active ingredients in the pills soon take their place in the landfill. Significantly, discarding medicine in the trash can also lead to the chemicals in the pills getting into the water supply. Landfills are often only a way station to water contamination.

Until 1937, when a bold idea was first tried in Fresno, California, there had been no facility anywhere in the U.S. that managed trash beyond collecting it and disposing of it by either incinerating it, sinking it in a large body of water, or, most commonly, leaving the garbage in an open-air lot that was usually called "the town dump."[47] Fresno's experiment changed the way that solid waste was managed. The idea there—since improved upon—was to compact the trash to save on space and to then apply a layer of soil to cover the refuse each day to cut down on rats, flies, and odors. As simple as it was, it was a revolutionary concept that was soon copied widely.[48]

Despite the improvement that the Fresno-style landfills offered over the then-common town dumps, they were still like those other helter-skelter scrap heaps in one important respect: The early landfills didn't address protecting groundwater. As the trash, aided by rainfall, would decompose, it would leach into the ground over where it had been placed. With little understanding of the geology of the sites where those landfills and dumps were located, yesterday's garbage became a future threat to that community's water supply. Over time, plumes of trash-residue-contaminated groundwater traveled to drinking water sources near and far. Because landfills and dumps were often placed over aquifers or in sandy areas over shallow water tables, contaminants of all kinds percolated into the groundwater.[49]

There are more than 1,800 active landfills in the U.S. today.[50] They are all subject to a variety of federal, state, and local laws and ordinances. Among these rules is the requirement to separate out any regulated toxic or radioactive material, and to dispose of it separately.[51] Another rule for active landfills requires sealing the bottom of the landfill to prevent leaking, and also to have a system to capture leaks when they do occur.[52]

Despite the current legal mandates for active landfills, one can assume more than a few failures of compliance. Since consumers can't be expected to know all of the categories and products that can be hazardous, it is a near certainty that some homeowners unknowingly mix benign-looking—but dangerous—substances with the many categories of trash taken to U.S. landfills.[53] Of course, it could also be that some people and businesses discard dangerous items deliberately, without concern as to the larger environmental consequences.[54] And the site itself may not always be built or managed exactly as required, especially given the economic incentives for fiscally strapped towns and cities to skimp on strict adherence to costly rules.

But even if all active sites were built and managed exactly as they should be, there are more than ten thousand landfills in the U.S. that were established before current regulations went into effect in the 1970s and are now closed.[55] These sites may be permeated with contaminants of which pharmaceutical residues are only one of many threats. Aside from yesterday's newspaper and the remains of last night's dinner, consumer trash often includes, to give only a very few examples to highlight the potential danger, fluorescent and low-power light bulbs containing mercury and other heavy metals, automotive products like car batteries, antifreeze, and fuel additives, and paint and paint thinners.[56] And, of course, unused medicines.

In addition to these municipal landfills, there are also as many as forty thousand other now-closed landfills of varying sizes that were created at industrial sites and in rural communities prior to the development of more protective standards.[57] Because these were used as a receptacle for a wide variety of uses, their now-capped contents present a variety of hazards.

As the array of discarded items in these many landfills break down over many years, chemicals flow from them in a liquid discharge that landfill engineers call "garbage soup." Unless a landfill was sealed before closure, this toxic broth presents a major threat to the current and future quality of groundwater. And even if properly sealed, utilizing all of the products and techniques required for doing so, it is, at best, a long but temporary stopgap. The materials used for sealing landfills are themselves likely to begin to degrade after thirty years—if not sooner—while a landfill can continue to emit a flow of dangerous chemicals for hundreds of years.[58]

Smaller in footprint than landfills, but far larger in distribution, septic systems are also a threat to groundwater. There are no federal regulations for septic systems, and the few state or local ones are focused on their initial installation, but not on subsequent testing for leaks and their environmental impact.[59] About a quarter of all Americans aren't hooked up to a sewage line of the kind that takes household sewage to a municipal treatment plant. For these 26 million American homes lacking such infrastructure, household sewage travels a short distance from the house to a septic system on the homeowners' property where the most basic, or primary, wastewater treatment takes place.[60] The more advanced secondary, or biological, treatment found now in nearly all municipal wastewater treatment plants is not a part of the septic system treatment. Despite their potential to pollute the groundwater around them and then far beyond, the EPA plays no role in overseeing or regulating America's vast network of septic systems. There is no federal regulation of private septic systems. Local enforcement is likewise difficult to manage, and spotty at best.[61]

The only time septic systems are sure to be tested after initial installation is if, when the house is subsequently purchased, the buyer applies for a mortgage. To obtain a mortgage, banks require that there is working sewage disposal for the home.[62] Other than that, a septic system can go a generation or longer without being checked, and even the mortgage investigation doesn't check for leaks.

Since septic systems, by design, drain the partially treated wastewater from the home's toilets, sinks, and showers, it isn't a surprise that even if the septic system doesn't leak, pharmaceutical residues and other contaminants that flow into them will eventually flow out of them, and then into the ground. Properly working septic systems aren't intended to provide advanced wastewater treatment, but even that basic treatment can be lacking. When a septic system leaks, as many do, that waste doesn't receive even the most basic treatment. Raw sewage streams into the groundwater.

Curious to see whether septic systems were a means of transmittal for more than nitrogen from human waste, in 2011 the U.S. Geological Survey (USGS) tested groundwater in Fire Island, New York, a summer resort community for many of the New York area's wealthy families as well as for up-and-coming singles piling into shared houses. In the groundwater surrounding the area's septic systems, researchers found hormones, detergent, insect repellent, sunscreen additives, floor cleaner, and a variety of pharmaceutical products.[63]

A more recent study in Cape Cod, a Massachusetts vacation mecca, demonstrates how pharmaceutical products escape untreated from septic systems where the contaminants then travel through groundwater, ending up in drinking water wells. In an area largely served by septic systems, the researchers examined twenty community wells serving the general population. Fifteen of them tested positive for contaminants of some kind, including suspected carcinogens, and in twelve of them some combination of antibiotics, hormones, blood pressure medication, prescription pain relievers, psychopharmacological drugs, and anticonvulsants were found.

Although none of the concentrations for these compounds exceeded current health guidelines, six of the eighteen contaminants that were tested for and found—including three for flame retardants—do not yet have established health standards. Further, the authors of the study noted the "limited understanding of low-dose exposures or interactions among multiple chemicals," suggesting that without much more research, there is no certainty that current health guidelines are necessarily the last word in the health threat from contaminants like these, and others, found in drinking water.[64]

All of those polluted wells were (and still are) in current use for drinking water. Because each of the contaminants found were at concentrations below a triggering violation, the utility that distributes the water is not out of compliance with EPA regulations. Under current law and regulation, the water is fit for consumption.

Aside from the "Yuck! Factor" reaction to such items in drinking water, the presence of these drugs and other contaminants in drinking water wells is cause for alarm, and not just for the people living or vacationing in Cape Cod or Fire Island. While septic systems are common in rural and poor parts of the country, Cape Cod and Fire Island are magnets for wealthy vacationers, people who may be accustomed to having—and who often demand—the best of everything. The local population in Cape Cod swells from 215,000 in the off-season to more than 500,000 each summer, and from 292 year-round locals on Fire Island to 20,000 in the hotter months. If the water supply in affluent playgrounds like these can become polluted with pharmaceutical products and other contaminants, it is logical to assume that the less economically well-off parts of America—many of which are serviced by septic systems—may also have toxic elements in their drinking water wells.

"Now We Know"

Whether from surface water or groundwater, it is now certain that pharmaceutical residues and more than a few chemicals are getting into our drinking water. Not every gulp, everywhere, but widespread enough that it should be a matter of concern to both the FDA and EPA. Both of these federal agencies should be testing for the presence of these contaminants and also their effect on human health.

While it isn't clear what the long-term consequences of these chemicals in our drinking water will be, common sense suggests that it would be wise to limit it or, if possible, to prevent it. The reason that prescriptions are required for every one of the thousands of FDA-approved drugs is because—if taken by the wrong person or taken in the wrong dosage or taken for the wrong duration—there is potential for harm. Yet, with bits of thousands of drugs in our drinking water, every one of us is at risk of taking sub-therapeutic doses, again, with unknown long-term consequences.

Professor Dror Avisar heads the Water Research Center at Israel's Tel Aviv University. His career-long academic and scientific efforts have been largely devoted to tracking contaminants in drinking water while also searching for chemical, biological, or physical technologies to render them harmless. Aside from his practical work in hydrochemistry, he is also something of a philosopher and futurist in the world of water.

"We know a lot more about water today than we did forty and fifty years ago when the last major round of wastewater treatment plants were being built," Avisar says. "But we shouldn't deceive ourselves that when these plants were built that there wasn't already chemical contamination in the water. We just didn't know about it, because we didn't have a way to measure it. It was there and it was entering the bloodstream of people, but we weren't able to act on it, because we didn't know enough about it. Now we know and the question is, 'What are we going to do about it?' We could close our eyes back then and pretend that everything was fine. But with what we know or what we are on the verge of knowing, we can ask different questions and come to new assumptions."

With water scarcity leading to growing amounts of water being re-used, Avisar says we have entered into a new era in history, one potentially as transformative for humankind as other major historical periods. "We have created the anthropogenic water cycle," he says. "For better and also for worse, rather than getting our water only from rain or from rivers or aquifers, now we are getting some or a lot of the water we drink from our own immediate recent use. With water scarcity more common and with growing populations a reality, the widespread reuse of water is a certainty. With that comes responsibility. If we are going to be reusing our drinking water over and over again as if we are on a space shuttle to Mars, we must be sure that that water is free of things that can harm us."[65]

But Avisar isn't an alarmist. "We know a lot more than we did just a few years ago, but we still don't know all we need to know," he says. Avisar proposes that, among other new kinds of research, drug testing of the type now being done by the FDA be transformed to include the new reality of minuscule doses of a variety of drugs being ingested by lots of others than that drug's target population. He believes that the more we know, the more the public will demand the purification of our wastewater and drinking water.

"I'd like to see drug testing required not only by the FDA, but also the EPA," Avisar says. "The FDA can test for its intended uses and the EPA in smaller, unintended doses. As part of that, we can see how each drug can be effectively neutralized or brought back to safe base elements so that wastewater treatment protects the public's health. A drug has a second life after it is used by the patient. The FDA protects that patient in the initial use. We need the EPA to protect everyone else for the subsequent use."[66]

Dr. Luke Iwanowicz, the USGS research biologist who studies, among other contaminants, the effect of estrogen on fish, explains how the FDA's comprehensive drug testing may have been less complete than imagined. Drug testing, he says, starts by wanting to know the toxic dose so that an upper limit for the drug may be set. Then, testing of ever-lower doses continues until the drug has no measurable effect on the subject.

"What we are beginning to understand," Iwanowicz says, "is that there may actually be an impact below 'No Effect.' . . . Ultra-low doses of estrogen, and also other drugs designed for a different purpose [that are getting into drinking water], could be causing hormonal disruption with effects on reproductive and sexual health, but from drug levels far lower than earlier imagined."[67]

Professor Diana Aga, the analytical chemist from SUNY Buffalo, also believes a rethinking of pharmaceutical products is necessary, and she has ideas on how to reduce the threat to public health in drinking water from them. "One of the reasons we have so much pharmaceutical residue in the water is because doctors may overprescribe drugs, more than what the body can absorb," Aga says. "Not everyone needs 400 milligrams of this and 25 milligrams of that. If we would right-size the prescription to the need, the patient wouldn't be taking more medicine than he or she needs and there would be that much less of the chemicals in the pills getting into the water. We could reduce the pollution load." Presumably the same would be true of veterinary drugs, which also contaminate our source water, especially because of the widespread dosing of otherwise healthy farm animals with hormones and antibiotics.[68]

Aside from right-sizing prescriptions based on body weight or other factors, Aga believes the pharmaceutical companies could do something even more significant. "It is still somewhat science fiction," she says, "but it isn't hard to imagine designing medicines so that their residues can be returned to their basic inert elements after they are used or that they become attractive to friendly bacteria which can break them down into something harmless. Many active ingredients in drugs are designed to be durable. Even after they are excreted, they persist in the environment."[69]

Nearly every scientist interviewed for this book shared the belief that wastewater and drinking water treatment should also include removal of pharmaceutical and other chemical residues. More than one said that it is only a matter of time before that becomes the norm. "These wastewater treatment facilities were created to remove nitrogen, phosphorus, and dissolved oxygen, and, by so doing, to reduce algal blooms," says Avisar using vocabulary similar to other scientists and hydrochemists interviewed. "But they were never focused on chemicals, in general, and pharmaceuticals, in particular."

The connection, he says, between the chemicals in water and a range of possible diseases and ailments had also mostly not yet been made. Now we know a lot and have the means to remove contaminants, whether in wastewater or drinking water, and in extraordinarily low concentrations, Avisar says.

The most common reason given for not requiring municipalities to upgrade their wastewater treatment plants—and drinking water plants, too—is the cost. This is why Avisar believes the best place to start is with the toxic wastewater at every hospital.[70] But he also thinks that the concern about cost may be looking at it the wrong way.

"When you discuss wastewater treatment just in terms of its raw cost," says Avisar, "it is quite expensive. But when you compare it with the cost of treating diseases created by ingesting the contaminated water or the cost of repairing or remediating polluted rivers or oceans, we could say that instead of spending a fortune on river and waterway rehabilitation, that we can spend some of it at the source. The question for every country is, 'What are your priorities?'"[71]

Five

PLASTIC EVERYWHERE

*"The chemicals in bottled water can be seen as a super cocktail.
It contains a bit of this and a bit of that. If one of them alone
isn't a hazard, we can't be sure what happens
when several chemicals in different amounts
are consumed together."*
—Professor Martin Wagner,
coauthor, *Freshwater Microplastics*

THE STONE AGE, Bronze Age, and Iron Age have been designated as the three great prehistoric and ancient eras of humankind. If a period can be defined by a transforming material, historians may someday refer to our era as the Plastics Age. But plastic isn't only the ever-present basis for most of our products. In one form or another, the chemicals used to make plastics and the residues from them are also found widely in drinking water, whether from the tap or from bottled water.

Plastic may be the most successful example ever of turning trash into gold. In its many forms, plastic used to be mostly derived from impurities removed from crude oil in the process of refining it into gasoline, diesel, or home heating oil. It is now produced either from crude oil or, more commonly, as a by-product of natural gas.[1] This "waste product" has evolved into a huge industry of its own. Of the $4.4 trillion in chemical sales worldwide, plastics are one of the largest segments, accounting for about $650 billion of that. In one form or another, plastic is found in more than seventy thousand products, and is used in industries as varied as automotive, packaging, computers, and aerospace, among many others.[2]

For both good and bad, the rise of plastic mirrors the importance of the crude oil and natural gas from which it is derived. Just as these carbon fuels grew to be of extraordinary value both for those who extract them and those who use them to power industry and the world's economies, plastic became a lucrative business while transforming global commerce. But while carbon fuels and plastic have led to countless benefits, in recent years those benefits have begun to be balanced by awareness of risks brought on by both.

Similar to the way in which oil and natural gas continue to be the world's dominant energy sources even as the dangers of these carbon fuels become apparent, there is no other material available today that can replace plastic. Indeed, efforts to create new kinds of plastic continue in laboratories around the world. Depending on what characteristics are sought—such as flexibility, durability, weight, or temperature sensitivity, to name a few—chemists have been able to arrange molecules to achieve a dizzying variety of alternatives. Nearly all of these familiar and new plastics have a related chemical structure, but each also has enough variability that the formulation results in a different product with unique properties.

Aside from the trash that so much plastic creates, there is another problem with some types of plastic. Most of the time, exposure to plastic is believed to be benign, or, at least, having no currently known ill effect. But some of the plastics, even a few in very widespread use, have consequences beyond polluted seas and litter-filled riverfronts. They also affect human health.

Unlike a stable material such as glass, when drinking water comes into contact with some finished plastic products, chemicals from the plastic can leach into the water. One widely reported example of this is Bisphenol A, which may be more widely known as BPA. This lab-made compound has a structure similar to a human hormone. As discussed in more detail below, when swallowed, BPA can create disruptions in the human endocrine system. In another instance, also discussed more fully below, vinyl chloride leaches out of PVC plastic, potentially causing impairment in the central nervous system. Vinyl chloride has also been confirmed as a human carcinogen.[3]

Knowing of the possibility that some plastic products can pose a public health threat to drinking water, it would be logical for there to be a process to research the potential harm before introduction of the product. This might be done in a modified version of the way in which the FDA demands pharmaceutical companies prove that proposed new drugs are safe for humans. Yet with plastic there is no such precautionary approach from the EPA, FDA, or any other government agency. The effect of the weaker-than-ideal controls on plastic (and other new chemicals) is that testing of these compounds gets done, but in a different way than anyone might want.

Dr. Shanna Swan, a professor and researcher at the Mount Sinai School of Medicine in New York, has spent her career studying the interface of synthetic chemicals from plastics and the ways in which they disrupt the human body's hormone-related activity. "Humans have become the guinea pigs to test the effect of new chemicals," she says. "These compounds get released without adequate testing, and five or ten years later we start to see cancers or hormonal disruption or infertility or other problems. That leads to research getting done that should have been conducted years earlier before the approval for release was given."

What ensues is what Swan describes as "an endless game of Whack-A-Mole," the children's activity where pushing a make-believe mole back into its hole only leads to another mole popping out of a different hole. In this real-world version of the game, chemicals come to market and, years later, when health concerns become suspected, a demand for testing begins. When the chemical is linked to a medical condition, the chemical companies often challenge the science used in the study or find other ways to keep sales of their product going for as long as possible. Then, says Swan, when consumer complaints start to be heard widely or political pressure starts to be felt, the company withdraws the chemical and re-sets the clock by introducing an "analog chemical" that has a similar chemical structure while technically being different. Because of that comparable chemical structure, the new compound offered as a replacement will likely cause the same or similar health problems as the withdrawn one it supplanted, but, as with its predecessor, the effects don't become apparent until several years after the "new" product has been introduced.[4]

None of this is a call to ban plastic. Just more than one hundred years since its first commercial use, plastic is the dominant material of our times. If one wanted to do so, it would be nearly impossible to go even a day without contact with it in some form. Yet even with a great appreciation for all of the ways in which plastic has improved our lives, a hanging question about plastic is: At what cost?

Is Bottled Water Safer than Tap Water?

America's bottled water industry achieved an important milestone in 2016. For the first time, the volume of bottled water sold in the U.S. was greater than that of carbonated and sweetened soft drinks, or what, depending upon the part of the country, is mostly called soda or pop.[5] The success of the bottled water companies—among whom are such beverage giants as Coca-Cola, which bottles and markets Dasani, and PepsiCo, which does the same with Aquafina—is all the more remarkable because of the disparity in what is spent in marketing in the two categories. For every dollar spent on bottled water advertising and promotion, the soda brands spend nearly thirty.[6]

Bottled water's success has less to do with marketing than with a change in popular attitudes. Consumers today buy bottled water for four main reasons: They prefer the taste, something that is of special value in places with local water that has high mineral content. They like the convenience of having water at hand along with the ease of being able to discard the container. They were or are soda drinkers but want to reduce or avoid consumption of sugary drinks to cut down on calories and to promote better health. Or they are afraid to drink tap water because of a concern it may be contaminated.[7] There is reason to believe that the last of these four is the most compelling.

In a November 2017 Harris Poll in which those questioned could list more than one reason as to why they drank bottled water, 99 percent cited "quality" and 92 percent "safety" as an explanation for their beverage choice. That those two attributes should rank so highly isn't a surprise when matched with consumer research from August 2015 that reported 60 percent of bottled water is consumed in the home.[8] Since tap water ordinarily flows freely there and is generally available for less than one-tenth of one percent of the cost of bottled water, consumer purchases are compelling evidence of people's priorities—and worries.[9]

That so many people should be fearful that the drinking water in their homes is unsafe should be of concern to every public official whose job touches on water infrastructure and the quality of what comes out of the tap. Every person who is drinking bottled water, especially when tap water is close at hand, is making a statement that government and the water utilities have failed to assure them that the available tap water is as clean, safe, and pure as bottled water is *perceived* as being.

While bottled water is often safer than tap water, the people driven to bottled water as a kind of immunity from contamination may not always be getting the level of purity they imagine. The nearly twenty pages of technical language in small print in the U.S. Code of Federal Regulations that addresses bottled water is mostly devoted to the acceptable limits of ninety-one contaminants, including coliform bacteria, arsenic, lead, and benzene, and how to test for them. This list confirms that—even if all limits are honored and even if, by being below those limits, the federal government says that the water is safe to drink—the water in that bottle may still contain contaminants that the consumer was not expecting.[10] Bottled water consumer information labels contain mostly worthless nutritional data like calories, fat, carbohydrates, and protein (all of which are zero), but carry no information about bacteria or chemicals that may be found in representative samples of the water.

As to which of the ninety-one regulated contaminants are found in any given bottle of water and at what levels, one scientifically rigorous study that tested at least three samples of more than one hundred bottled water brands revealed that the presence and mixture of contaminants is nearly as broad as the number of bottled water brands that were tested. In all, about one-third of the brands examined had at least one sample that exceeded recommended levels for bacteria and/or chemical contaminants. The researchers also found little uniformity, with the quality of the water often varying for the same brand of bottled water from one production run to the next. Different contaminants at different volumes were found in different samples from the same brand. Some of those individual brands that had an excess of contaminants in one sample showed no trace of those same impurities in other bottles tested.[11]

There are at least seven hundred brands of bottled water in the U.S., and one industry expert says there are probably far more than that.[12] While a few water brands are nationally famous, many companies take advantage of the very low barriers to entry into the marketplace and have one or more bottled water labels that they use on water sourced and filled from the same location. Many regional and local bottled water companies aren't brands for which their owners invest in enhancing consumer awareness as much as they are easily forgettable—and replaceable—trade names. As might be expected, these many marketers of generic bottled water generate little or no consumer loyalty. Their sales are driven mostly by their depth of distribution and (low) price. The lack of consumer connection allows the "brand" to disappear and then for the same water to reappear under another name.

Some of the bottled water products come from protected springs or other natural sources as is the case with Perrier, Evian, and Fiji. Yet others of the bottled waters started as tap water, but are then enhanced and significantly purified, as are Dasani and Aquafina. And some of the bottled water on the market is not much more than tap water put into a bottle with all of the contaminants that may be in that water remaining. Because of a lack of controls on branding and labeling, as long as bottled water marketers don't make false claims as to source or health benefits, their products can be presented with descriptive or fanciful names and with illustrations that imply a connection to nature and purity.

But even without making explicit claims of superiority in healthfulness and cleanliness, the subliminal message of the bottled water industry is that tap water isn't safe and, by implication, that the implied purity of bottled water provides better long-term health prospects. Paradoxically, despite the popular perception of the greater safety of bottled water over tap water, bottled water is subject to even less government supervision than the water we get in our homes.

Unlike tap water, which comes via pipes from a municipal water utility and is regulated by the EPA, bottled water is under the supervision of the Food and Drug Administration (FDA). As poorly resourced as the EPA drinking water regulatory and enforcement effort is, the FDA's is even more so. Despite the billions of dollars in sales of bottled water each year in the U.S., and despite its widespread consumption, the FDA has no institutional structure akin to an Office of Bottled Water. Considering that the bottled water industry generates $18.5 billion in annual wholesale sales in the U.S., and, on average, every American consumes forty-two gallons of bottled water each year, you might think there would be a large staff at the FDA devoted to bottled water. But, there isn't.[13] The FDA has two employees who work on bottled water, and both of them also have non-water-related responsibilities.[14]

As a result, the federal oversight of bottled water in the U.S. is barely a step up from a self-policing honor system. Despite that lack of oversight, large companies with established brands have a lot to lose financially and risk damage to their reputations if people get sick from their water. To avoid even a remote possibility of that, these large companies make quality control and adherence to regulatory requirements core concerns and build the competencies necessary in order to prevent bad publicity or, worse, a recall. Testing to assure that bacteria levels are harmless and that contaminants that are required to be measured are all within federal, state, and industry limits becomes part of regular practice.[15] Nestlé, for example, owns many familiar water brands, including S.Pellegrino, Poland Spring, Arrowhead, Deer Park, Calistoga, Ice Mountain, and Zephyrhills, among others. The Swiss food giant also owns and markets a filtered tap water brand called Nestlé Pure Life. Quality in all of those can't be guaranteed, but each brand benefits from parent company oversight and expertise.

Even for multinational corporations in the water business—and certainly for the no-name brands—being in full compliance with the law does not mean the water is as pure as might be imagined or desired. Bottled water needs only to be below the maximum levels of the ninety-one bottled water contaminants set by federal regulation. The water in those bottles doesn't need to be contaminant-free as their labels might imply, or as consumers might assume.[16]

More concerning is that, by volume, most of the bottled water sold in the U.S. isn't required to follow FDA bottled water guidelines at all, even as limited as they may be. If water is bottled and sold within the same state, it is exempt from FDA regulation. That leaves it to each state to establish rules and to monitor those bottled water companies that are exempt from FDA oversight doing business exclusively within its borders. If a state adopts the federal regulations or has a significantly staffed department to oversee bottled water quality and compliance, it is a benefit to consumers. But no state is obliged to do so, and many don't.[17] Since more than 70 percent of all bottled water distributed in the U.S. is both bottled and sold in the same state, there is a lot of bottled water consumed that does not have federal oversight and isn't required to adhere to any federal regulations.[18]

America's Favorite Beverage, 70 Billion Times a Year

Consumers seeking safer drinking water may often be right to think bottled water is the better alternative, but they can't always be certain they have made the right choice. For sure, by one measure, bottled water is safer than tap water. In more than twenty years, there have been only six bottled water product recalls, and in a recent five-year period studied, there were no reported cases of bacteria-borne illness from bottled water. By contrast, even accounting for the fact that the national tap water system is far larger and serves more people than those who get their drinking water from bottled water sources, each year there are more than two thousand Boil Water Alerts issued for when excessive amounts of bacteria get into the drinking water supply. It is also confirmed that several million Americans get sick from tap water every year.[19]

Bottled water's record of apparent hygienic success may be misleading. It may be due to the modest amount of supervision by the FDA and state agencies, resulting in a failure to detect violations. Or it may be because the private-sector-driven, self-policing model of the bottled water industry works well. But the general absence of sickness-inducing bacteria in bottled water isn't enough to say for sure that that water is healthier. Without a lot more supervision and testing, it is hard to be certain.

What is certain is that consumers yearn for safer, purer water, and that they are prepared to pay a large price premium over the cost of tap water to get that peace of mind. Although reasons for its appeal vary, approximately one-third of all Americans drink bottled water on a regular basis, and more than 60 percent identify still or sparkling bottled water as their favorite beverage.[20] Perhaps there is a message in that for government officials who could charge a very little bit more for tap water and deliver far better quality. If tap water offered all of the real or perceived advantages of bottled water, it is worth asking if millions of people would pay what amounts to hundreds (and often thousands) of times more for a bottle of water than for the same volume of water they could get from the tap for less than a penny a day.[21]

Other than advertising and marketing expenses, and beyond allowing for profit, the explanation for why bottled water is sold at such a premium over tap water varies. The water may need to be transported from far away, as with Fiji water, bottled in pristine conditions in the South Pacific, and then shipped thousands of miles.[22] Other brands, including Dasani and Aquafina, go through advanced treatment, such as reverse osmosis that is able to remove contaminants down to extraordinarily low trace levels, rendering the water as pure as any drinking water likely to be found.[23] Other bottled water companies need to purchase or rent the (mostly) uncontaminated springs from which their water is drawn, or distill the water before bottling it.[24] In each of these cases, the water in the bottle is likely to be purer than what the consumer will get from no-name local bottled water, and possibly also from tap water.

Since the 1977 U.S. introduction of Perrier, a naturally carbonated spring water sold in France since 1898, sales of bottled water have grown meteorically in America, compounding year after year with growth curves rarely enjoyed by any consumer product over a sustained period. Perrier helped to create a consumer category thanks, in part, to marketing its product in distinctive green glass bottles. As the bottled water category grew, other brands preferred the lower shipping costs of plastic containers, with the implied purity of water that could be seen through the clear plastic as an added benefit. Today, less than 2 percent of bottled water comes in glass of any color, and in 2002 even Perrier switched distribution and sale of its non-restaurant bottled water to (green) plastic containers.[25]

All of that convenient, lightweight plastic comes with consequences. While the implication of so many plastic water bottles on trash disposal and landfills have been discussed often, a topic of less public awareness is what effect that plastic bottle may have on the health of the person drinking from it.[26]

One health concern is that disposable plastic water bottles can be a source of phthalates for those drinking from them. Phthalates (pronounced THA-lates) are a chemical that have been shown to interfere with the body's hormonal system. They can block production of androgen, a male hormone that, among other functions, produces testosterone. While the threat to men, boys, and male fetuses seems most obvious, phthalates can cause hormonal disruption in women and girls, as well.[27]

Phthalates were first introduced in the 1920s, and have long been added to a wide range of plastic products like shower curtains, vinyl floor tiles, and plastic food packaging. They are also used in the manufacture of the plastics used in disposable plastic water bottles and their more rigid caps. The caps are made of either polyethylene or polypropylene, and are a confirmed (minor) source of phthalates. A different plastic—polyethylene terephthalate, or PET—is used in the manufacture of disposable water bottles. They often have residues of phthalates after their manufacture. Even more concerning, bottles stored for long periods or kept in hot places, such as outdoors or in a car during the summer, are even more prone to have phthalates migrate from the bottle into the water.[28] Since it is usually impossible to know how plastic bottles were warehoused prior to sale, no one knows the risk of drinking from any particular PET water bottle.

While one disposable water bottle may look like the next, from a chemical point of view, there are differences. With 70 billion disposable drinking water bottles sold—and discarded—each year, no one chemical company could supply all of the raw ingredients, or resin, needed.[29] More important, there is no precise consistency in the chemical makeup of the resin feedstock needed to make the PET bottle from one supplier to the next and, at times, even from one shipment to the next by that same supplier. From one batch to the next, the raw ingredients usually differ. Because of this, the chemicals in one production run of PET bottles will almost certainly differ from another.

Professor Martin Wagner, a biologist with a special expertise on the effect of plastics on the human hormonal system, believes that there is a greater potential threat to public health from the unknown elements in resin feedstock than there may be from phthalates. "Producers of PET bottles and other plastics aren't forthcoming about what chemicals are in their raw materials," says Wagner. "They may not even know. But there are many possible combinations of chemicals in plastic packaging, and some of them may be toxic." What isn't always certain is whether dangerous chemicals will be found in any given bottle, and, if so, which ones and at what levels of concentration. Without industry standards and adequate testing, no one can know for sure.

But based on recent research he has done, Wagner has reason for concern. Using a sophisticated, state-of-the-art mass spectrometer that can report the presence of chemicals at even trace levels, Wagner has found some disturbing results, especially for those who turn to bottled water in the hope of getting pure water. Without exception, in every bottle tested, chemicals of some kind were found. Whether that was from the source water used to fill the bottle or from chemicals leaching *from* the plastic *into* the bottle, Wagner's investigation couldn't determine.[30] But in all of the bottled water samples put through the spectrometer, the chemical "fingerprints" of at least nine hundred compounds were found, even if often at ultralow concentrations.[31]

"The chemicals in bottled water can be seen as a super cocktail," says Wagner. "It contains a bit of this and a bit of that. If one of them alone isn't a hazard, we can't be sure what happens when several chemicals in different amounts are consumed together."[32] As with other researchers in this growing field of toxicology, Wagner calls for a lot more testing.

Water Bottles and "Regrettable Substitutions"

Perhaps the most notorious example of contaminated water that came from a plastic-related source was the reusable, durable plastic water bottle popular with students and sports enthusiasts. For many of them, they began using this bottle in an attempt to reduce the volume of disposable plastic. But unbeknownst to these environmentally sensitive consumers, a chemical called Bisphenol A, or BPA, was leaching into the water in their bottles.[33] Because BPA has a chemical structure similar to human hormones, it can disrupt endocrine systems, especially in fetuses and newborns.

Even an effort by these well-meaning people to stay completely away from plastic—reusable or disposable—was to no avail. BPA wasn't limited to plastic bottles. To prevent corrosion and avoid a metallic taste, manufacturers of metal water bottles usually lined the inside of their bottles with BPA. Whether as a reusable plastic bottle or as a liner for a metal one, BPA was getting into the drinking water of millions.

In September 2008, the National Institutes of Health issued a report expressing concern that BPA could be an endocrine disruptor, with effects on the brain, behavior, and prostate gland of fetuses, infants, and children at current levels of human exposure.[34] Further investigation expanded the circle of those who might be harmed. Research demonstrated that BPA—which is toxic even at very low doses—could result in, among other adverse outcomes, severe birth defects, including abnormally sized and shaped male or female genitals in newborns and a much greater chance of being infertile in adulthood.[35] More recent studies have also linked BPA exposure to accelerated puberty, and to increased risk for cancer, heart disease, and diabetes.[36]

An outcry by consumers led to the FDA banning BPA baby bottles and sippy cups in 2008, but not sports bottles. Acting where the FDA did not, thirteen states and the District of Columbia later banned BPA sports bottles and use of BPA as a liner inside cans of baby formula. This resulted in manufacturers halting production of BPA water bottles, and soon thereafter affixing "BPA-Free" labels on the products manufactured to replace the now discarded original BPA bottles.

Unfortunately, the BPA-free stamp on the new reusable water bottles was likely more of a marketing tool to calm frightened users of their products than it was a bona fide public health notice showing concern. What consumers buying replacement water bottles labeled as being BPA-free almost certainly did not realize was that most bottle manufacturers had replaced the BPA they had been using with a near-exact chemical copy called Bisphenol S, or BPS.[37] Technically, the BPA-free claim was truthful. But as regards to the implied lack of potential harm from their new water bottles, only time will tell.

The BPS substitute for BPA is an example of what the Mount Sinai School of Medicine's Professor Shanna Swan calls an "analog chemical," or what others call a "regrettable substitution." It took many years to conclude that BPA is an endocrine disruptor.[38] With BPS, the chemical companies producing it and the manufacturers using it get a do-over. But given the history of BPA, it would be a good idea—and a valuable precedent—for the EPA to test BPS *before* allowing it to be adopted widely for drinking bottles. But that isn't the way the system works. At least, not yet.

Plastic Pipes and Leaching Contaminants

Plastic comes together with drinking water in more than just different kinds of bottles. Mostly for reasons of cost, many municipalities and home builders have begun using different kinds of plastic pipes to either replace failing metal pipes or in developing water distribution networks for new buildings and neighborhoods.

One of the plastic pipes commonly used is polyvinyl chloride, or PVC. PVC is derived from the chemical vinyl chloride. During the PVC manufacturing process, it is common for some of the vinyl chloride to fail to be converted into plastic. The unconverted vinyl chloride remains embedded in the PVC. When the PVC comes into contact with water flowing through the pipe, some of the embedded vinyl chloride leaches into the water. When ingested, vinyl chloride can affect the central nervous system with symptoms including dizziness, headache, fatigue, and even loss of consciousness. Vinyl chloride has been definitively linked to liver cancer, and, as mentioned earlier, is one of a limited number of chemicals that U.S. officials have concluded should be classified as a "known human carcinogen."[39]

The amount of vinyl chloride that will leach into the passing water will vary depending on the specifications of the manufacturing process used as well as the volume, temperature, and speed of the water that flows through the pipe. In the first three to six months of use, the quantity of vinyl chloride that leaches into the drinking water is considered to be at its peak, but some amount of vinyl chloride will continue to leach for, at a minimum, several years, even if at lessening volumes over time.[40]

Andrew J. Whelton is a professor of engineering at Purdue University and among the nation's foremost experts on the use of plastic in infrastructure generally, and in water distribution systems in particular. More than a high-tech plumber, Professor Whelton's academic concerns center on the interaction of plastic infrastructure and human health.

"PVC pipe is only one of several kinds of plastic pipes being installed to distribute water," Whelton says, mentioning several others in a rapid-fire list. "If there is a common element about all of them, it is that there has been inadequate research about their short-and long-term leaching. There is no review by the EPA of plastic pipes."

He points out an inconsistency in the government's approach to product safety. "There is the federal Consumer Product Safety Commission [CPSC] that compiles data and issues safety rulings on thousands of products. In another product area like pharmaceuticals, the FDA demands that data must be kept and shared. But for the plastic pipes that drinking water flows through, there is no formal system. The limited information available has been developed by a handful of [academic] researchers."

Even this research is constrained by a professor's ability to get funding for his or her work. When the research grant runs out, investigation into the plastic pipes and the amount of leaching stops. In any event, Whelton says, "New products are introduced faster than we can ask questions about them. When poorly performing products are discovered, unlike with the CPSC, there are no nationwide recalls."

Whelton says that he and other academic researchers face the same reaction that health and safety advocates experience in other industries when health concerns are disclosed about their products. "The manufacturers and the plastic pipe groups have big budgets and can deploy them to question the validity of any new study," he says. "In the meantime, the plastic pipe companies are selling plastic pipes every month without regard for the cost of possibly having to dig them up later because of health concerns."

Another plastic pipe being increasingly used in water distribution also poses a health concern that Whelton believes is under-researched even as its use continues to grow. An epoxy-based resin, Whelton explains, is inserted in failing water mains, lead service lines, and building plumbing, and it is then heated. After it fills in spots where there is a crack, the resin cools and hardens. The repaired pipe remains in the ground or behind a wall in a home or building. This saves on the cost of removing the damaged pipe and on purchasing and installing a new one. What the public in those towns and cities using this epoxy-based resin likely doesn't know is that it is another form of BPA plastic, the same material that is now banned for use in baby sippy cups and shunned by runners and other athletes for their water bottles. Whether it should be banned in water mains, too, Whelton can only say that it should be independently researched before billions of dollars of the epoxy-based resin is installed.[41]

Whelton points out that some testing and certification on plastic pipes is done, but it isn't by the FDA, EPA, CPSC, or any other federal agency. The only entity that tests plastic pipes, he says, is NSF International. Especially in drinking water safety, those are easy initials to confuse. Here, "NSF" doesn't stand for the National Science Foundation, which is an independent scientific agency of the federal government, but, rather, for what used to be called the National Sanitation Foundation, now rebranded as NSF International. Although the Michigan-based organization is a not-for-profit entity, it accepts payment from the pipe manufacturers whose products it tests, which may reasonably leave room for questions about objectivity.[42]

Even if a plastic pipe has received an NSF International seal of approval, it doesn't speak to its safety in drinking water. Due to inconsistencies in the manufacturing process, the same type of product installed in a home may differ chemically from the one that was tested. And even with the modest amount of testing of a specific kind of plastic pipe, there are no standards to assure that a pipe that has been approved by NSF International for drinking water will be used by a contractor for that purpose or if another plastic pipe will be substituted.

"Your health is at greater risk," says Whelton, "because plumbing design has not kept up with technology advances—and people think that everything is okay."[43]

Whelton calls for more data sharing and transparency by industry to allow independent researchers to piggyback on their research. "It isn't clear," he says, "if [the plastic pipe] industry knows what and how much their products leach. There is no law or regulation requiring them to test their products or to test at the tap in people's homes, and there's no law requiring them to disclose what they know." Further, Whelton says, if one of the pipe manufacturers is sued and data was developed for the litigation, when they settle the case the parties agree to seal court records and the public can't get access to that information.

"Everything is kept behind a veil," Whelton says. "The public is kept in the dark."[44]

Plastic Everywhere, Smaller than the Eye Can See

Among the enduring photos that helped to launch and sustain the environmental movement are those of a river on fire, immobilized sea birds covered with oil from a petroleum tanker spill, and shorelines of lakes and rivers covered with rotting fish killed by toxic chemicals.[45] Each of these was proof of the natural world run amok due to human carelessness or overreach. If rivers on fire or mass kills of fish and birds in waterways are less common now thanks to laws demanding better practices, today's shocking online videos are of waves of plastic debris washing onto beaches.

The idea of us swimming in a sea of plastic, it turns out, is less a metaphor than might have been realized only a few years ago. Around the year 2000, oceanographers, marine biologists, chemists, and other scientists came to note an alarming trend. Lots of plastic was in the world's oceans, and thanks to ever more precise measuring instruments, it was possible to start taking account of plastic found there in tiny pieces unseen by the human eye.

In 2016, the world produced about 335 million tons of plastic, an amount that grows each year.[46] Only about 10 percent of that gets recycled, while about half of the plastic manufactured becomes trash within a year.[47] According to a recent academic study, because of dumping, littering, or poorly maintained landfills, somewhere between 5 and 13 million tons of plastic got into the oceans in 2010 alone, a total annual volume nearly certain to have increased since that research report was completed.[48]

Once in the ocean, the plastic doesn't become reduced. Rather, it changes form. Plastic is mostly made of carbon compounds that reflect its origins from crude oil or natural gas, but it may also have hydrogen, oxygen, nitrogen, chlorine, or sulfur, among other components.[49] In a perfect world, plastic would be returned to those base elements in a process called mineralization. Instead, because plastic is so durable, it doesn't degrade. Instead, it breaks down into ever smaller pieces, many with a diameter of less than a millimeter, or what is less than 1/25th of an inch. These ultra-small plastic disks are called microplastics.

In addition to plastic trash that breaks down into very small pieces, beginning in the late 1990s cosmetics and personal care companies began adding pieces of plastic called microbeads—each less than a millimeter—to shampoos, soaps, toothpaste, and other products, supposedly to enhance performance. These microbeads were washed down the drain and were so small that only a few U.S. municipal wastewater treatment plants had (or have) the means to filter them out of the sewage in the way that larger pieces of plastic and other debris are removed. When the treated wastewater is discharged from the facility, the billions of microbeads that survived the treatment process were deposited into a receiving

body of water. The environmental threat of microbeads led to an international movement to ban their use in personal care products. Even
with the U.S., in 2015, being among the first to ban it, this novelty will
leave a long legacy.[50] Since microbeads are made of highly durable plastics like polyethylene and polystyrene, they will be in waterways for a
long time to come.

Added to the large amount of plastic packaging and microbeads, there
are other forms of plastic also barely visible to the naked eye. There are
several thousand chemical combinations of what are called man-made fibers, the most famous of which is polyester. These fibers also get washed
down the drain and, as with microbeads, are too small to be captured
by screens and filters at most wastewater treatment plants. Likewise, car
tires are made of a plastic synthetic chemical. As they wear away, tiny
bits of the tires are found on highways and roadways. When rain comes,
these synthetic plastic bits are washed away, ultimately into a waterway.[51]

A few years ago, a relative handful of enterprising scientists began asking if the presence of these different forms of microplastics found so
widely in the world's oceans might also be present in freshwater. If so,
they wondered, what was its effect on our drinking water and our health?
Their hunch that microplastics weren't just a problem for the world's
oceans was correct. All of these—the degraded plastic packaging, the
microbeads, the synthetic fibers used for clothing, the worn-off pieces
of tires, and more—find their way into rivers and lakes, many of which
are also a source of drinking water.

Just as chemical contaminants of many types are found in both tap
water and bottled water, microplastics are found in both of them, as well.
Research done in 2018 that surveyed thirty-three tap water samples from
around the U.S. found microplastics in all but one. The average number
of plastic particles found in these samples was nine pieces, with one
sample yielding sixty-one plastic fibers or fragments. That same research
also tested bottled water from around the world. Three bottles of American bottled waters were tested—not a large sample, but microplastics
were found in all three.[52] Although possibly less relevant to the U.S., a

German study of twenty-two glass and plastic bottles of water done at about the same time found microplastics in every one of those sampled.[53]

Because freshwater is a central ingredient in many other products and because the significant majority of drinking water filtration facilities are not currently designed to trap and remove plastic particles of that size, it isn't a surprise that microplastics have also been found embedded in a variety of products manufactured with drinking water. The same researchers who did the tap water study examined twelve samples of beer brewed with water from each of the five Great Lakes. In each sample and regardless of which lake was the source of the water, microplastics were found.[54]

As research into microplastics accelerates, we can expect to find these tiny bits of plastic elsewhere. Microplastic contamination of food from all of the plastics used in the preparation and packaging have been confirmed.[55] And with water being a part of nearly everything that is produced, and especially so for processed food and beverages, it, too, can be a source. With drinking water drawn from source water likely contaminated with microplastics and with only a very few drinking water distribution facilities anywhere adequately screening out microplastics from tap water, consumption of these tiny pieces of plastic is now likely a near-universal experience for Americans and for others living in industrial societies.

Putting aside the "Yuck! Factor" of eating, drinking, even inhaling these bits of plastic, the key question that will drive solutions to this problem is whether microplastics are a danger to human health. Some small marine creatures have starved due to misidentifying the plastic bits as a food source.[56] Certainly, no comparable risk is likely for humans. We consume lots of indigestible, and at times even jagged, items that our bodies pass from our system. Still, it would be worthwhile to know more about the long-term effect of human engagement with these plastic fragments. As with much else involving contaminants that have found their way into drinking water, we are playing catch-up. Our level of understanding isn't equal to the volume of plastic all around us.

Professor Martin Wagner is among a small group of young academics who have done the leading research into the emerging field of microplastics in freshwater. "We have a legacy of billions of tons of plastic in the environment," he says. "If this very afternoon, an invention came out that would allow us to never use plastic again, plastics would still be around for long time. We make plastic to last, and it will last for decades, maybe even centuries."

Wagner is impatient, eager to change the status quo as it relates to plastics. "We need to change all of this. We need to begin designing plastic so that it is safe for humans and safe for the environment. The chemical companies that are designing plastics should be talking to toxicologists and environmental scientists, rather than waiting until the product has been manufactured and sold, and discovered to be a problem."[57]

"This Problem Just Can't Be Overstated"

Veena Singla is an expert on how chemicals in the environment affect people. In her work at University of California, San Francisco, Dr. Singla examines connections between everyday products that contaminate our water, air, food, and soil, and the impact of that contamination on human health, especially reproductive health. She has also analyzed federal legislation for the EPA and has prepared technical proposals for chemical risk evaluation that the environmental agency might follow.[58] From both her scientific and policy perspectives, she has concluded that the regulatory system doesn't fit the needs of the times in which we live.

"A doctor or a scientific researcher," she says, "would always demand to prove that an item is safe first before it is introduced for widespread use. But that isn't what we do. Instead, we allow chemicals to be introduced, and only after they have been used by people for several years do we determine if they are hazardous. Instead of doing testing in a controlled laboratory setting, we are testing products and the chemicals in them on broad population groups. That isn't the announced policy, but functionally, that is what's happening." Singla acknowledges that this is how chemicals and products have always been introduced in the U.S., but says, "This approach may never have made sense, but especially not now."

The "now" that Dr. Singla speaks of is the post–World War II era, and especially the past twenty years. "In one public health issue after another," she says, "the problem can be traced back to the explosive growth of the use of plastic. It is hard to overestimate this effect." Instead of addressing specific chemicals used in the production of plastic that have become recognized or suspected health hazards, Singla speaks, in a general sense, of what she calls "the life cycle of a product," and the several points during which contamination may occur.

She starts at the point of manufacture. "When plastics are manufactured," she says, "the water and air around the factory get contaminated. But the contamination often travels via air currents and water flows, and sometimes very great distances." Then the product goes into use. It may be something disposable or it may be something like a computer with a plastic casing or a sofa with synthetic textiles that stay in your home for many years, but either way, in most cases there is an ongoing leaking of chemicals into the air from those plastics. The chemical released as a gas may land on food or glasses of beverages and be consumed. Babies may crawl on a carpet and get chemical residue on their hands and then put it in their mouths. Or the chemicals that leak from the plastics in your home may get into air currents and later land on surface water.

"That water may be source water for drinking," Singla says. "Or fish may ingest the chemicals and then be eaten by humans. But either way, the chemicals can end up being consumed by people."

The final stage of the life cycle that Singla describes is when the products are discarded. They go to a landfill and, she says, over time, unless the landfill is perfectly sealed, the chemicals in them leak into the groundwater there.

"From beginning to its end, the circle of contamination is wider than most people imagine," she says.

As concerning as this life cycle may be, Singla has a yet deeper worry. While some chemicals degrade and break down over time, many of these are designed to be exceptionally durable. Also, some chemicals get into the body and then get flushed out, but others don't. "There are several persistent, bioaccumulative chemicals that just build up in our bodies," she says. "It's hard to know what the long-term health effects of these chemicals are, but it is possible to say that some of these are cancer risks, and also risks to human endocrine systems and reproductive health."

Beyond the science, Singla also addresses policy and politics. She cites the power of the chemical industry over legislation and in blocking solutions. "This problem just can't be overstated," she says. "Unlike some issues that ebb and flow with the politics of the day, the lack of oversight [on control of chemical contamination] is felt regardless of the party in power in Congress or the person in the White House."[59]

There is, she says, an imbalance between the power of industry, and its ability to pour money into campaign donations and lobbying efforts, and the power of the public interest groups to protect against the sale of potentially hazardous chemicals. "The public is larger, but the chemical companies are better organized," she says. "Until the public gets organized and demands laws that can protect our health, the imbalance in power and outcomes will continue."

Singla says we need far more testing, better scientific insight, better policies, and better laws. "Chemicals," she says, "don't just magically appear, and they won't just magically disappear."[60]

Six

ONE CITY OF MANY: FLINT AND LEAD IN AMERICA'S DRINKING WATER

"It is a lot of little lies that add up to one big lie."
—Professor Marc Edwards,
water resources engineer

FAIRLY OR NOT, Flint, Michigan, is now thought of as the place where everything fell apart. Even if you know almost nothing about drinking water in America, you likely know the name Flint, and connect it to unsafe water. The question about Flint is whether what happened there was a one-of-kind, never-before-and-never-again story, or whether what occurred in Flint is repeating itself, undetected, in other towns and cities across the nation.

The answer may be both.

It is hard to imagine that the long chain of management failures and ignored safeguards could be duplicated elsewhere as dramatically as happened in Flint. But the inadequate required monitoring, manipulated testing, falsified results, poorly trained staff, outdated facilities, and the consequent contamination of drinking water—from lead and other sources—that was found in Flint is also present to some degree in many other cities. Compounding this breach in consumer safety and public health, many water utilities, municipalities, states, and even the EPA are complicit in these negligent or reckless practices.

How Flint's lead crisis began is without dispute. The city had collapsed economically. Over several decades, about half of its population had left and the 100,000 or so who remained behind were, mostly, poorer people who didn't have other options. Management of Flint got put in the hands of the state, and officials appointed a manager in September 2013 to "right-size" the city's budget. As part of his work, the manager looked for expenses that could be reduced or eliminated.

Until that cost-cutting exercise began, Flint had long gotten its water from Detroit's water utility, about seventy miles from Flint. Detroit sourced its water from Lake Huron, one of the Great Lakes, and before distributing the water—whether to Detroit's homes or to Flint—Detroit's water utility "polished" the water by adding what are called anticorrosion chemicals to it. These chemicals build up a film on the interior walls of lead drinking water pipes with the purpose of creating a separation between the lead surface of the pipe and the water that flows through it. Without that separation, the lead in the pipe leaches into the water as it comes into direct contact. To save on costs, in April 2014, the Flint manager decided to replace the supply of the Detroit water with a less expensive alternative from the nearby Flint River.

Inexplicably, in making the transition, the Flint water utility failed to test the acidity and chemical properties of the Flint River water, which, as it turned out, had a composition very different from that of the water in Lake Huron. Whereas the Lake Huron water was compatible with the anticorrosion coating that had been built up on Flint's pipes, the Flint River water was highly corrosive. While skilled engineers at a well-run water utility would likely have been able to manage the difference in acidity between the two water sources, the staff at the Flint facility lacked adequate training to address the different water chemistry.

In addition, because of concerns about the Flint River's cleanliness, the river water required anti-pathogen treatment. In yet another error, although the cleansing agent selected was the same as the one used in Detroit, the Flint utility decided to increase the amount used without noticing that, at the level applied, it was also highly corrosive.

While the addition of anticorrosion chemicals may sound mechanical and the creation of the protective barrier inside the pipes fairly easy to achieve, they aren't. Anticorrosion treatment requires a degree of technical sophistication that isn't available for all of the public water systems in the U.S. The amount and type of chemicals needed to be added to get that inner lining—to, in a sense, paint the inside of the pipes—varies considerably based upon the ever-changing acidity of the water, its mineral content, temperature, the water pressure in the pipes, and other factors.

As just one example of those many other factors, in the days and weeks that follow a snowfall and the spreading of rock salt on highways, the salinity of river water rises—and so does the water that flows into drinking water treatment plants. Along with the other variables mentioned, the higher salinity has to be taken into account in managing and treating the water supply. But with each change, the corrosion control chemicals being used need to be modified flawlessly, and sometimes quickly, to prevent the pipes from being stripped of their protective inner layer.

When the Greek philosopher Heraclitus wrote that a person can't step into the same river twice, he meant it as an insight about how life changes as quickly as the water in a river flows. But his statement is also correct from the perspective of water chemistry. Water may seem the same, and certainly so in the same body of water, but it often isn't. And with the switch to Flint River water and the high volume of cleansing agent being added, the anticorrosion layer in Flint's pipes was stripped away. Soon, the lead in the pipes connected to about fifteen thousand homes became exposed.

Without warning to the people of Flint, lead levels in the city's drinking water began rising in the months following the April 2014 switch to Flint River water.[1] When rashes and other ailments were reported, Flint residents were told by local and state officials that the cause couldn't be the city's water because the water was safe, even healthy. Government spokespeople shared results from recently taken lead testing. These statements confirmed that the people of Flint had nothing to worry about, that lead levels were low.

Yet, despite the reassuring statements, the opposite was true.[2]

A Problem of Unknown Scope

Consumption of any amount of lead presents a danger, with fetuses, babies, and young children suffering the most immediate effects. But the lifelong impairment isn't only felt by them, even if primarily so. Society at large also suffers. In the best case, when a potentially smart person is exposed to lead, it drops an otherwise high-IQ person down a few points, depriving society of a potential special achiever.[3] At its worst, though, lead fouls a young person's neurological system, and drives down intelligence and social abilities, setting the person up for a lifetime of needlessly missed opportunities.

Because of the then rapidly developing brain, the most damage done by lead is in the prenatal period and during the first five years of life. Exposure to lead during that time not only can result in delayed development and impaired social engagement—think of a baby smiling when eye contact is made—but also to lifelong deficits in basic cognitive skills like vocabulary acquisition and the ability to do simple arithmetic. Without significant and costly special education classes, tutoring, and other interventions, the effect of lead on children is both enduring and irreversible.[4]

In addition to lowering IQ, lead contamination can have a range of other health effects. In adults, for example, exposure to lead is known as a cause of miscarriages and male infertility. It can also lead to high blood pressure and heart disease, and from those, elevated rates of cardiovascular deaths.[5] Even brief exposure to lead can result in fatigue, headaches, insomnia, and a range of stomach conditions.

While the harm created by lead is beyond debate, what isn't known is the scope of the problem. Estimates of how many homes get drinking water that passes through lead pipes range from a low of 6.1 million to over 10 million, with an unknown number of people and children in those households.[6] Those numbers rise when other lead plumbing sources are added. People are also at risk if they live in homes that have pipes with lead solder used to close joints, or water meters or shut-off valves with lead interiors. Even galvanized steel pipes can have built-up lead deposits on their interior walls. Indeed, unless you live in a home built since 2014 when federal laws banned use of lead pipes and have your water distributed from your community's drinking water plant with all new pipes, plumbing products, and water meters, you could be drinking water that contains lead.[7]

Homes aside, there is also a lead problem in many of America's schools and day care centers. Those school buildings (and also churches and other institutions that house day care facilities) that were built with lead pipes and components may also be putting an unknown number of children at risk.[8] One reason that the number of schools and day care centers with possible lead contamination isn't known is because a 1988 law mandating testing in both was poorly drafted. In 1996, a federal court declared the law unconstitutional on a technicality.[9] Although it could do so, Congress has not passed a successor bill amending the drafting error, but rather repealed the mandatory testing provision and replaced it with voluntary testing that schools and day care centers are free to ignore.[10] In the meantime, sampling tests at many public schools—in some cases required by individual states—have found a significant and widespread presence of lead in the drinking water there.[11]

Whatever the actual number of homes, schools, day care centers, office buildings, hospitals, and others affected, it is a certainty that the total comes to a large number. The total of those who are at risk of getting lead in their water is no fewer than tens of millions of Americans.[12]

A Protective Coating That May Not Protect

The lead problem became so vast because of practical and economic reasons. For as long as water has traveled through pipes, and especially since the 1880s when citywide piping of water by municipal water departments became commonplace, both plumbers and engineers have been partial to lead due to several special properties.[13] Most notably, lead is both flexible and more durable than other materials that can be used for distributing water.

That lead can be easily molded is important given the way that plumbing systems are designed. Water mains—the big pipes that bring water from a central distribution point—tend to travel in a straight path. They are very rarely, if ever, made of lead or lead components.[14] In contrast, service lines—the pipes that branch off a water main to bring water to a home—are likely to bend this way and that to get around obstacles and into the home. Once inside a home, pipes have to reach many rooms, and a straight path is impossible. Each turn requires elbows, sleeves, joints, and other plumbing hardware, and each connection needs to be sealed.

To address the winding and irregular infrastructure of pipes and connectors, lead's flexibility made it easy for plumbers to do their job. Lead solder was used universally to seal connections. Engineers also proposed the use of lead pipes and fittings because the metal doesn't rust or corrode. The interior walls of a lead pipe don't get thin, and pinhole leaks that are common with copper and copper-alloy pipes don't occur. Despite lead being more expensive than steel or other pipes, lead pipes were a better investment for municipalities and building owners because they lasted so much longer.

Unlike other metals, lead doesn't decay from contact with soil. Since service lines are always placed underground, whether for short or longer distances, lead pipes are perfect for conveying water from the water main to the house. With the average lead service line rarely shorter than 25 feet, and some as long as 160 feet, there is potentially a lot of lead surface area to come into contact with drinking water as it enters millions of American homes.

By 1900, twenty-three of the twenty-five largest U.S. cities, and 85 percent of all cities, were primarily using lead service lines.[15] In recognition of its long life when buried, many cities made the use of lead pipes mandatory, at least through the 1950s, and in some cities, such as Chicago, for decades after that. Like other types of pipes, lead service lines were effective in conveying water, but lead also allowed municipal governments to not inconvenience their taxpayers (and voters) by having to dig up streets and sidewalks.[16] Those benefits, however, come with a continuing consequence. Although there are other sources of lead contamination from plumbing infrastructure, a 2008 study revealed that as much as 75 percent of the total mass of lead measured in tap water comes from lead service lines.[17]

Only during the World War II years, when lead production was diverted from pipes to make bullets, did the rate of lead service line installation slow. Right after the war, it bounced back to ever-higher levels of usage with the postwar boom. Returning soldiers starting families, and moving into new homes and communities, almost certainly were being supplied water from lead pipes or pipes sealed with lead solder, or both. Well into the 1980s, brass fixtures containing lead and a combination of lead and tin solder used to seal joints remained in common use in household plumbing systems.

Despite the benefits of using lead, the popularity of the metal through the first eight decades of the twentieth century is puzzling. Confirmation that lead might cause cognitive impairment in children first came in 1943. A psychologist-physician team working in Boston noted intellectual deficit in children with elevated levels of lead in their blood.[18] Evidence continued to grow in the following decades until the extent of the potential harm became more completely understood.

For example, beginning in the late 1970s, pioneering social scientist Herbert Needleman studied the long-term effects of lead contamination on children and found that those with high lead levels in early childhood had a seven times greater risk of dropping out of high school than those with low levels. Making the study even more surprising, the children with high lead levels came from more affluent families, and the control group, it was discovered later, came mostly from lower-income ones. This unexpected discovery demonstrated that, even with socioeconomic advantage, lead contamination is a powerful predictor of academic failure.[19] Other research by Needleman found that, regardless of race, family income, or the number of parents present in the household, young men aged twelve to eighteen years old with elevated lead levels were four times more likely to be arrested than a similar control group.[20]

But long before Needleman's path-breaking work, lead from drinking water was understood as a public health menace. In 1900, researchers in Massachusetts did a study of more than twenty municipalities with lead service lines. They found a direct correlation between higher levels of acidity in drinking water and a greater incidence of miscarriages, stillbirths, and infertility. Baffled by this at first, the researchers came to realize that the higher acidity had stripped away any mineral deposits that might have built up on the interior walls of the lead pipes. Without that mineral interface between the lead and the water, more lead was leaching into the drinking water. Simultaneously, these researchers also found that people in communities with high mineral content in the water—even when the acidity was also high—suffered relatively fewer of these and other conditions because, as they later learned, less of the lead was exposed because of buildup of minerals on the inside of the pipe.[21]

Despite the growing realization that lead pipes might be a cause of many different health problems, their use continued to proliferate in growing U.S. cities. Places with low levels of water acidity weren't immune from lead contamination. They only suffered less or felt the effects more slowly. The same was true for towns and cities with naturally high mineral content, as the minerals would adhere to the inner walls of the pipes and offer protection from the lead.

Professor Werner Troesken, in his fascinating 2006 historical work *The Great Lead Water Pipe Disaster,* points to a broad inclination of early-

twentieth-century municipalities and utilities to find ways to continue
to use lead pipes, and not to replace them. Some municipalities and utilities did all they could to address the problems lead pipes seemed to
create, while others ignored them. But one overriding idea adopted
everywhere lead pipes had been laid—likely derived from the seeming
immunity that communities with high-mineral content water enjoyed—
was to figure out a way to line the insides of lead pipes. The lining, it
was thought, would provide protection while still getting the other
benefits that lead's malleability and durability provide.[22]

Different communities tried different approaches in developing this
interior sheath. Ironically, the anticorrosion chemicals that proved to be
most effective utilized lead-based compounds such as lead carbonate or
lead phosphate to coat the inside of the pipes.

In 1991, more than fifty years after the first of these anticorrosion
efforts, the EPA issued the Lead and Copper Rule.[23] Rather than advocating for a twenty-year national effort to identify the location of and to
remove all lead pipes and plumbing fixtures as some had suggested (and
which would, in a perfect world, have been the best decision for the nation's health), the rule tried to institutionalize practices then in effect at
leading water utilities. Chief among them, the rule encouraged the use
of "corrosion control" to make better coatings in every lead drinking
water pipe's interior walls.

As a protective measure, and when it works properly, corrosion control can be effective in reducing lead content in water. But corrosion control does not entirely prevent lead in drinking water, and, at times, it
can even elevate the lead level significantly.[24] Low-frequency vibrations
can cause bits of the pipes' interior coating to come off. For example, if
there are vibrations from a passing truck or from roadwork, they can
shake the pipes enough to disturb the protective coating. And since most
of the anticorrosion coatings come from lead-based compounds, should
any part of the coating get shaken off, it can result in very high lead
levels.

One EPA official who lives in Chicago and whose work centers on lead experienced the hazards of this firsthand. When the street in front of his home was being opened a few years ago as part of a citywide water-main-replacement program, he became concerned that the vibrations could be shaking loose the lead-based coating inside the lead service line that feeds water into his home. He took samples of his tap water and sent them to a professor friend to test in his laboratory. His fears were confirmed, but to a degree that left even him—an expert in water-based lead contamination—dumbstruck. The lab tests showed a presence of lead of 455,000 parts per billion, thousands of times higher than the 15 parts per billion level at which the EPA demands action be taken.[25] Presumably, his neighbors in the same Chicago neighborhood were getting similar levels of lead contamination, but without having any idea that they should be concerned or needed to modify the use of their tap water.

Acting as a private citizen, even if one very knowledgeable about lead and lead pipes, the EPA official notified the city and told people in the Chicago water department that they should inform everyone whose street was being opened for new water mains. Whether the city sent out notices isn't clear, but the EPA official never received one at his home and never heard any news of it at the EPA's Chicago office.

No one on that street or elsewhere in Chicago or anywhere whose drinking water was being contaminated by lead would have any reason to know that they might have grossly elevated lead levels in their tap water. No matter how high the level of contamination, you don't taste, smell, or see lead that is in drinking water. Unlike with many other contaminants, boiling the water might even concentrate the lead, making exposure worse if the water is ingested as a beverage or used to cook food. Without testing, you wouldn't know you have a lead contamination problem until after you start to have physical symptoms from it. But such readily observable symptoms usually only occur after very high levels of exposure. At lower levels, though, lead contamination can be insidious. Because impacts from lesser amounts of lead contamination are subtle and hard to connect to drinking water, people may suffer from

IQ loss, miscarriages, fertility problems, or high blood pressure and cardiovascular disease without realizing the cause.

Determining those elevated lead levels is even harder than imagined: The testing for lead—*as designed by the EPA*—is so flawed that most of the time the results are wrong, misleading, or an invitation to the local water utility to commit fraud.

Cheaters Prosper

Mike Schock began his postgraduate career at the EPA in 1978, and has been a chemist on its staff for most of the last forty-plus years. Although not on the faculty of a university, Schock is the author or coauthor of more than two hundred scholarly articles, most of which are studies of the interaction between water and lead-containing materials. It is no wonder that he is believed to be one of the most knowledgeable scientists working in the field of lead and drinking water.

"Lead," says Schock, "is a different kind of problem than other contaminants in water, and needs to be addressed differently. Different samples from the same faucet taken a few moments apart can show variability [of lead] from very low to very high and then back to low. Or very high to moderate to low to high. That's because lead is not uniformly distributed in the water the way most other contaminants are."

In the case of all other regulated contaminants, the local water utility is obliged to neutralize or filter the contaminant at the central water distribution center down to the EPA-established safe level *before* the water leaves the facility. Because lead gets into the water long after it is gone from the water utility's facilities, with rare exceptions lead contamination can't be treated at the source.

Since testing for lead at the drinking water distribution facility is of little value, it makes it all the more urgent that accurate testing be done at places where the threat of lead contamination is likely or possible. Not only is that important for the health of individuals, but without proper data collection, developing macro solutions for communities and the nation becomes all the more difficult.

As Schock points out, the same faucet can provide several different lead readings over the course of only a few minutes. One myth he is eager to dismiss is that a family can protect itself from lead contamination by allowing the water to run for a minute before drinking from that tap. This so-called "flushing of the line" may work, but without knowing the location of the lead pipes feeding the house, it is impossible to be sure. Even though drinking water professionals know that how you sample for lead will affect what you find, Schock says, testing of the entire flow from tap to the water main is almost never done. Likewise, Schock adds that "sampling of tap water when it is being drawn for actual cooking, drinking, or beverage preparation" is a rarity.[26]

Research shows that the EPA's lead testing protocol, which calls for those performing tests to collect a sample by filling a single one-liter bottle from a kitchen or bathroom tap that hasn't been used for at least six hours, may not produce results representing either the exposure of the individuals in the house or the peak risk of lead in the drinking water at that location.[27] If a house is fed by a lead service line, "the 'first liter out' testing protocol will rarely produce a high lead level from water drawn that way," Schock says.[28]

Given the health consequences of lead contamination and lead's widespread presence, it would be fair to assume that EPA-mandated lead monitoring is ongoing and done with scientific rigor. But in practice, depending on a matrix of requirements, cities test their water for lead only every six months, every year, or every three years. The mandatory home sampling ranges from five to—even in a metropolis like New York City or Boston—a maximum of one hundred. Generally, the samples are taken by ordinary residents without supervision.[29] Each of the houses selected for the test is supposed to be in a place where the likelihood of lead contamination is high, but there is no formal process for their selection. Participants in the tests are given a single one-liter bottle and provided with written instructions on how to fill it. Samples are to be taken just once, and then handed in.

As insignificant as the amount of testing done may be, there is another, more systemic, problem with the tests: They are done long after contaminated water may have been consumed. In most other cases in which a water utility is required to screen for regulated contaminants, the testing and treatment is done *before* the drinking water is distributed to the community. With lead, contamination could be occurring for as much as several years before a problem is detected. During that time, a large number of people—pregnant women and small children included—could be exposed to lead in their drinking water. Nothing need be done until *after* what is called an "action level" is reached.[30]

An action level is determined by using a mechanical formula. After a community has taken the samples obliged to be collected—whether five or one hundred, or some number in between—the test results are arranged in order of the lowest amount of lead concentration found to the highest. If the sample that is at the 90th percentage point—say, the second highest concentration of ten samples—is higher than 15 parts per billion, an action level is declared. This does not result in a fine or a penalty of any kind. The water utility is required to give notice to the community and to take steps to enhance corrosion control. The utility is also expected to take action by removing some lead service lines.

Even if every testing requirement were scrupulously adhered to, the opportunity for error would be large. Yet, as bad as that would be, in many cases the reality is worse. There is widespread gaming of the testing system, often amounting to cheating and outright fraud. A few examples give a sense of the problem.

First, the water utility may fail to test enough samples, or to test at all, or to use only samples that have come in at a low lead concentration number. Second, the utility may select homes that are in neighborhoods more likely to report low lead levels or lead levels at zero. Third, since the amount of lead found is affected by whether the collection bottle has a wide neck or a narrow one, and whether the water runs directly into the bottle or at an angle, results can be manipulated by the materials distributed to those few people selected for testing. Finally, test results can be intentionally misreported or go unreported. Since there is either no penalty or, at worst, a modest one for failure to report, any utility that finds itself over the action level threshold can simply fail to report, choosing a modest non-reporting penalty from the EPA over the significant expense of corrective measures. Similarly, while some of the testing methods that can minimize lead detection noted here are either not allowed by EPA rules or are discouraged, the likelihood of getting caught and fined is infinitesimally small.

"The falsification of test results—and not just for lead—is an open scandal," says one water industry veteran who would only speak without attribution. "If you know where to look for it," he says, "you can find cheating. But the EPA hardly ever looks for it."

Lead testing, he says, is supposed to seek out homes most likely to have a problem, but those in charge of picking the participants in the test often do the opposite, or just add a few high-lead-profile homes, while still making sure that the testing doesn't trigger the need to take action.[31] Because of the honor system inherent in the way reporting is done—water utilities give data to the states and the states then turn the data over to the EPA—the utilities can provide whatever numbers they want. Bureaucrats in state agencies have little interest in getting into an argument with local communities, especially as the vast majority of water utilities are under the control of a local elected official.

Further, says the water industry veteran, few states have well-funded water departments to monitor compliance. This makes it easy for water utilities to cheat, but even when everyone is providing accurate information, the understaffed state water departments may take months before test results are reviewed and analyzed, if in fact they ever are. Without prompt review and analysis, the state isn't alerted to the presence of potentially high lead levels that might require action. "The next round of testing could be three years later," he says. "Individuals and whole

communities can be exposed to high levels of lead during this time."
And if bad results are suppressed, it will be even longer that dangerous
levels of exposure will continue without notice to those at risk.

A recent report stated that as many as thirty-three U.S. cities, including Chicago, Boston, and Philadelphia, manipulate lead testing to obtain more favorable results.[32] Another report said that it was standard
practice for "every major city" east of the Mississippi River (where lead
service lines are most common) to falsify the amount of lead found in
testing samples.[33]

Whether the testing is for lead or some other regulated contaminant,
"you can get any results you want and report any results you want," says
the industry veteran. "It is how Flint was able to file reports showing no
lead problem."[34]

Everyday Heroes, and Models of Activism

For the year or so when Flint was front-page news, it was easy to feel a
sense of despair. A poor, majority-black U.S. city had contaminated
water, and no one seemed to take responsibility. Even if the children living there had had perfectly safe water, they would be starting life at a
disadvantage. Add in the IQ-lowering and health-impairing effect of the
lead contamination they had endured, and you could feel yourself witness to the tragedy of lives being cut short in years or opportunities, even
before they had a chance to get going. With those impediments, the cycle of poverty and dependency would continue for at least another generation there. If people are cynical about government and other American
institutions, Flint was—at least, at first—all the reason anyone would
need.

But in a saga filled with incompetence, cowardice, bureaucracy, and
fraud, there are also points of light and inspiration. Several people stand
out as models of what can be achieved in repairing America's drinking
water. A seemingly immovable system can be moved. Ordinary citizens,

college professors, even lifelong government employees all helped to get Flint noticed when all everyone in power seemed to want was for the problem to go away.

LeeAnne Walters had a mother's instinct that the assurances from city and state officials that Flint's water was safe weren't correct. After some complaining to Flint's City Council, a city employee came to her home three times and tested her water on each visit. Although she wasn't told this at the time, the highest of the tests found the lead levels from her tap water at 707 parts per billion, nearly 50 times higher than the EPA's 15 parts per billion action level. The city only told her the result of the lowest test at 107 parts per billion (seven times the action level), but explained that since there was no problem with Flint's water, the problem must be in the plumbing in her own home. That, she was told, wasn't within the purview of the city, and was a problem that she would have to address on her own.[35]

Skeptical that she was getting accurate information, and worried about her four young children, Walters contacted the regional EPA office in Chicago. Her concerns got passed along to Miguel Del Toral, an EPA drinking water regulations manager, who thought something sounded amiss. On his own initiative—and breaking with standard protocol, which required him to refer Walters's complaints back to the state drinking water administrator—he decided to look into her complaint himself.

Although a more than four-hour drive from Chicago, Del Toral visited Flint twice, and then wrote a memo that laid out the technical cause of the problem. His memo detailed serial failures by Flint to adequately protect against lead contamination of drinking water. He also noted the significant rise in blood lead levels in the Walters children, and that it coincided with the changes in Flint's change of source water. Del Toral proposed solutions that wouldn't be implemented in time for those children, but which might protect others.[36]

In June 2015, at Walters's request, Del Toral gave a copy of his memo to her. She shared it with the American Civil Liberties Union (ACLU), and they, in turn, gave it to the Natural Resources Defense Council (NRDC). On behalf of the people of Flint, in January 2016, the NRDC and the ACLU filed a lawsuit against the State of Michigan and state-appointed Flint officials. The following January, the two advocacy organizations also filed a separate class action suit against the EPA on behalf of 1,700 Flint residents. The lawsuits claimed that the state and the EPA had failed to act in a timely way in addressing the lead problem, resulting in a public health crisis.[37]

Government bureaucrats are supposed to follow rules and not to develop their own procedures. Following Del Toral giving his memo to Walters but before the lawsuits had been filed, he was told by an EPA ethics lawyer to not speak to anyone in Flint or about Flint—or he would be at risk of violating unspecified EPA ethics rules. It was clear that following this advice would mean he could no longer assist Walters or help address the now obvious threat to public health in Flint. Although Del Toral was near retirement following his long career at the EPA and not eager to jeopardize his pension, he believed he had a duty as a public servant to help Walters and the people of Flint. He decided to ignore the "advice" and to continue providing counsel to Walters and others. Despite the implied threat in the instructions given to him, no action was taken by the EPA against Del Toral.

The class action lawsuit was settled in March 2017. The state government agreed to pay about $100 million to remove lead service lines across the city and to provide bottled water and water filters until that task was completed. All eighteen thousand lead service lines (and galvanized steel pipes likely to contain lead) were required to be removed and new pipes installed.[38]

Del Toral's writing and sharing of the memo that he prepared for EPA's management about Flint played an important part in setting in motion the events that would result in the replacement of that city's lead pipes. But it wasn't his only action that got Flint the attention it needed. Del Toral was also responsible for getting the most important lead pipe activist in the U.S. to become involved in the effort.

Soon after giving Walters a copy of his memo, Del Toral suggested that she contact Marc Edwards, a professor of environmental and water resources engineering at Virginia Tech. She did. No one did more than Edwards to make everyone aware of Flint's lead pipes, or to get Flint on the road to a new beginning.

A Courageous Advocate for Public Health

It doesn't take more than a few moments with Marc Edwards to understand that he isn't interested in making friends. He's prepared to be ostracized and alone. Indeed, Edwards doesn't hesitate to point fingers at people and institutions in the world of drinking water who he believes have failed society—even when he has a long-standing relationship with them. Showing no mercy or fatigue in his relentless attacks, he's not someone you want to have as an adversary. His accusations don't just sting. They burn.

One admiring professional colleague of his said of Edwards, "By nature, Marc is quiet, even shy. But he's seen so many lies told to protect the status quo that he's learned the only way to break through and protect people is by being aggressive and, sometimes, incendiary. He's prepared to do whatever it takes to get his point heard and to get action."

In 2003, Edwards was a young engineering professor hired for a routine consulting project by Washington, D.C.'s, water system. Leaks were popping up in the city's copper pipes, and as a subject matter expert, the local utility—which reports to the EPA—wanted Edwards's opinion as to the possible cause. Although outside of the precise mandate of his assignment, Edwards decided to test Washington's water for lead. He was astonished by what he found. Lead levels were, he says, "outrageously high."[39] He began to investigate.

The professor soon figured out what no one else had noticed. The city had changed from using a simple chlorine chemical to purify the city's drinking water to a different chlorine-based compound. Although the new chemical did as expected in neutralizing dangerous pathogens and keeping the community safe from waterborne bacteria, it was also highly corrosive to the protective material that had built up on the inside of the lead pipes. The compound, he realized, was stripping off the protective layer that years of anticorrosion chemicals had added to the inside walls of the city's lead pipes. The lead was now exposed to the water in the pipes, and Washington's 23,000 lead service lines had become conduits for lead leaching into the water.[40] As a result, Edwards found that lead levels in drinking water were very significantly above the EPA's own 15 parts per billion action level.

When Edwards raised the matter with the water utility, instead of it choosing to investigate, he learned that his contract had been terminated. Efforts to get the EPA involved resulted in his being shut out from other consulting assignments by the federal environmental agency. When he attempted to continue the research on his own time, both refused to share data about lead or anything else with him. He was persona non grata.[41]

Edwards didn't live in Washington, and the lead in the water didn't affect him or anyone he knew. Faced with a situation like this, most young professors eager to have a consulting practice to augment their academic salaries would probably forgo challenging the EPA and the D.C. utility, and leave it to others to make major policy decisions. But rather than meekly retreat in the face of such powerful institutions, Edwards says he became obsessed with the possible implications for the children of Washington, D.C. Wanting to know if the limited data he had found would prove to be broadly accurate, he took out a mortgage on his house to finance testing of the tap water of individual homeowners in Washington and also to pay for filing Freedom of Information Act requests to regain access to the information he would need to make his case.

A year later, with data in hand, Edwards concluded that there had been widespread lead contamination of Washington's water, something never reflected in the test results filed by the utility with the EPA. When confronted by him, neither the EPA nor the D.C. utility would concede an error had been made or that changes were urgently needed. Worse, the EPA brought in the Centers for Disease Control and Prevention (CDC)—the most important public health agency of the U.S. government—to analyze Edwards's claims. Edwards believes that the EPA asked the CDC to issue a report rebutting them, which they did.[42]

Edwards spent the next six years fighting the false impression that he had fabricated a health emergency. Working on his adopted cause to the exclusion of other assignments, he lost years of opportunities to earn consulting fees. In the long process fighting for the children of Washington, D.C., Edwards spent more than $100,000 of his own money, plus all of the $500,000 he received from a MacArthur "Genius" Prize in 2007.[43] His tireless advocacy led to a congressional investigation, which in 2010 vindicated him.[44] The CDC was forced to issue a retraction.[45]

With the bruising Edwards got from the long fight, he might have been entitled to let someone else be responsible for getting Flint's situation addressed. But after being contacted by LeeAnn Walters at the EPA's Miguel Del Toral's suggestion, once again Edwards jumped into action.

Edwards faced the EPA and the State of Michigan, which, based upon the tests that had been filed, believed all was well in Flint. Edwards again threw himself into his new cause. And again, he used his own money—this time, $150,000 over several months—to finance waves of students to drive the 550 miles from Edwards's Virginia Tech campus to Flint where they could properly test the local water for lead.[46] With Edwards putting his name and reputation on the line and with the data developed from his testing, Flint got attention and became the model for what must be done when water is suspected of being contaminated. But had Edwards not succeeded in Washington, it is fair to assume that there would have been no one with enough credibility to put Flint on the national agenda.

For Edwards, Flint was a great success, at least when compared to Washington. "The people of Flint got safe bottled water to drink. They are getting their [lead] pipes replaced. The children are getting tutoring and help. None of this should ever have happened," he says, "but at least there was action taken. The children of Washington, D.C., never got help."

What also kept Edwards from being able to get allies in his Washington struggle, he believes, was that government bodies tend to support each other rather than looking out for the public they are created to serve. Although he stops short of calling for privatization of all of the country's water systems, Edwards says, "The irony is that if all of the water systems in America weren't government owned, we would have fixed this long ago. The government would never have allowed the private sector to get away with creating this kind of harm. We would have a program to replace all of the lead service lines around the country, and we'd demand honesty in testing."

Regardless of who owns or runs the nation's water utilities and regardless of who appoints the EPA's and other senior government officials, what is essential for Edwards is a change in mindset. "We have to stop allowing people in positions of power and authority to look the other way when there is dishonesty in the water testing. It sends a message that a corrupt culture is okay. Once people get away with it once, they do it again and again. It is a lot of little lies that add up to one big lie. And," says Edwards, "it's a lot of little unethical actions that add up to poisoning the children."[47]

Cities Working Against the Public Interest

Winston Smith (not his real name) is a current senior EPA official. Because of what he described as his agency's cumbersome approval process for allowing professional staff to speak with the media, he asked to not be identified so that he could speak freely. He wanted to share what he considered to be important, but not widely known, information.

Smith is a believer in total lead pipe replacement. As with others interviewed, he points out the scope of the problem, the lack of public awareness, and the quiet opposition of mayors and other elected officials to launching a bold effort at getting the problem solved. Where it works, he supports the use of corrosion control, but its effectiveness can't always be assured, he says, because of the complexity of the process and the lack of properly trained staff at many water utilities.

"A major impediment to getting this problem resolved," Smith says, "is that in some major cities, it would take ripping up one street after the next to get the lead out. You have to have the public ready for that kind of disruption, and most mayors aren't doing what they should to explain why it is needed. On top of that, some cities actually put up impediments to their people replacing their lead pipes."

Take Chicago as an example, and not a random one. While Flint had fifteen thousand lead service lines at the start of the crisis before an aggressive replacement program began, Chicago alone has as many as 380,000 such pipes that need replacement. Contributing to the difficulty of removing such a large number of pipes, Smith says, it is yet harder because of a variety of policies that Chicago—but not only Chicago—has in regards to removal of lead service lines.

If you live in Chicago and want to replace the lead pipe into your home, Smith says, the city charges an assortment of fees totaling more than $3,000. Driving expenses higher, Chicago city government requires all lead service line replacements to be handled by someone who is a member of, what Smith describes as, "the politically powerful local plumbers' union." While Smith concedes that it makes sense to have licensed plumbers handle lead service line replacements, this arrangement works against the public policy goal of getting lead pipes removed. Including the city's fees, the total cost of lead service line replacement in Chicago ranges from $15,000 to $20,000 per pipe. "These charges," Smith says, "compare unfavorably with some U.S. cities that have successfully replaced their lead pipes for a total cost of as little as $3,000 per pipe."

Chicago's policies are the subject of special ire by Smith. "On top of all of these fees and roadblocks, from the 1880s to 1986," Smith says, "Chicago made the use of lead service lines mandatory. Given the health consequences that follow, it would be fair to expect the city to take some responsibility for its ill-fated decision to compel lead pipes and to do all it can to assist those of its residents interested in removing them."

But Chicago isn't the only big city with a lead service line problem. Smith believes that New York City may have a worse problem than Chicago. "Not only is corrosion control erratic in New York City," he says, "but the city has fobbed off responsibility for most of the lead service lines there on other people and businesses. The city says that its responsibility ends with the water mains. Because the city says the service lines aren't theirs, and because most homeowners and landlords who have lead service lines likely don't even know that their properties have them, no one is taking responsibility. Meanwhile, while this is being allowed to continue, New Yorkers are being kept in the dark."

In January 2019, a few months after the interview with Smith, New York City announced a campaign to make the entire city lead free within ten years. The ambitious effort states an aspiration to replace all lead service lines as well as to remove lead paint in apartments and lead found in soil in the city. Even cosmetics and other personal care products that contain lead would be restricted.

The best guess is that there are 130,000 lead service lines in New York City, but no one knows for sure. Lead pipes were regularly connected to brownstones and small apartment buildings through 1961. Patch repairs on lead service lines were permitted as recently as 2009. But city records didn't always indicate what kind of metal was used in an installation or a repair of a service line. Yet whatever the correct number, the official announcement of the program makes clear that the city government doesn't see it as its responsibility to remove all of them. Pointedly, in the materials issued for the announcement of the program, the lead pipes are referred to as "privately owned."[48]

Starting with a pilot program that would pay the costs of replacing 1,900 lead service lines for low-income, single-family homeowners, the hope is that the program will expand, and that as water mains are replaced, landlords will use the opportunity to also replace the lead service lines into their buildings. The city is budgeting about $2,700 per line replacement. If extrapolated citywide to replace all of the lead pipes, the cost would come to a bit more than $350 million over ten years, but with the majority of that being paid for by property owners.

New York's mayor, Bill de Blasio, said in a recent interview that despite the modest start to this program, he is eager to see it result in complete lead service line replacement. "The only acceptable number of children exposed to lead in New York is zero," he says. He also expresses a hope that the New York program will inspire other cities. "We are a leader in many areas. I'd like for us to be a leader here, too."[49]

"This Is a Problem That Can Be Solved"

Getting rid of the lead in America's drinking water won't be easy, but it is achievable. Because of the size of the problem, and the expense and inconvenience that will be incurred in solving or reducing it, few public officials are eager to take it on. But where cities have made it a priority, like Lansing, the capital of Michigan, or Madison, the capital of Wisconsin, all lead service lines were replaced in under ten years.

Hank Habicht has a special vantage point from which to comment on the steps needed to develop a national program of lead pipe removal. During the administration of George H. W. Bush, Habicht served as the EPA's deputy administrator, the agency's number 2 position. His duties included overseeing the EPA's lead policymaking. In 1991, after intensive internal study and technical analysis, the EPA's Lead and Copper Rule was announced. Although the rule did not make total lead replacement its primary approach, it was generally supportive of it. Instead, the rule placed emphasis on enhanced testing and corrosion control, making it obligatory wherever lead pipes were found.

With the perspective of more than a quarter century, Habicht says that, "The view then was that corrosion control might be able to solve the problem, and at far lower cost and inconvenience than total replacement. In practice, corrosion control has helped bring down total lead levels considerably, but implementation has been uneven. Therefore, now may be the moment to begin advocating for total replacement."

Habicht offers a few ideas on how to get there. "Around the country, there is growing recognition that safe water infrastructure is essential for both the health of the community and its businesses," he says. "This awareness needs to be encouraged. As momentum to modernize our water infrastructure builds, complete lead pipe replacement should be a key part of the agenda."

To achieve this, Habicht says, "We have to educate the public about the risks of lead that they and their neighbors are incurring. Once the public decides that this is something important to them and to the well-being of their communities, there will be the political will to solve the lead problem once and for all. For now though, most mayors are reluctant to be in front on this, and that will continue until they know that the public is prepared for some extra expenses and some inconvenience like tearing up streets and front yards. But public education, and from that an engaged public, is the key."

Even so, Habicht doesn't make an all-or-nothing argument. Referencing Flint and other places where the public wasn't protected, Habicht says that until all lead pipes are removed, corrosion control and other treatments must be properly and transparently implemented. Beyond corrosion control and even before total replacement begins, he wants to be sure that several steps are taken.

"We need to be sure that we don't make the situation worse than it already is. It is essential to make sure that no new products that contain lead are used in drinking water systems." In support of this, Habicht proposes training municipal plumbing inspectors to play an expanded role in public health.

"If it is known that projects and repairs won't get approved if plumbing components that leach lead are found," Habicht says, "contractors and plumbers will quickly stop using them."

Another step he proposes would be to mandate that plumbing products bear identifying marks to show that they are certified to be lead-free or resistant to lead leaching. "That," he says, "would make it easy for consumers, contractors, and plumbing inspectors to avoid lead products."

Habicht also thinks that real estate brokers and home inspectors can be made a part of the nation's public health infrastructure. Just as they are now obliged to see if a home has lead paint, realtors and home inspectors can be asked to check if the home's water comes via lead service lines or faucets and valves containing lead. Where pipes can't be seen, he says, home inspectors can be trained in how to do testing.

"All of this must be handled cost-effectively and in a way that respects the privacy of the owner of the house," Habicht says. "If lead pipe disclosure was developed into a selling point, homeowners would be motivated to replace lead pipes while they are readying their home for sale. Ideally, they would receive financial benefits or incentives for doing so." Lead-free homes, he says, could be of special interest for families with young children.

Habicht also offers some nontechnical advice. "Although it is tempting to do so," he says, "it is important to not go looking for someone to blame. That will put mayors and others into a defensive mode and will only delay building support and finding solutions. Let's all agree that today's lead problem is a legacy of an earlier era when there was incomplete information and build from there. If we didn't fix this in the past, let's move beyond that and resolve to take on this challenge now. This is a problem that can be solved."[50]

Seven

THE WATER INDUSTRY

"People think that water is simple,
but it is highly complicated."
—David LaFrance,
CEO, American Water Works Association

A MERICA'S DRINKING WATER institutions and the physical infrastructure they oversee are both in need of an overhaul. More than one million miles of aged water mains transport the country's drinking water, with at least 240,000 of these pipes breaking every year. Much of this vast system will need to be replaced in the coming years. Finding the money and the labor to do this will be challenging, especially as no one has been saving up for this inevitable day.

As hard as it will be to repair and replace this physical infrastructure, it will be yet harder because of America's water utilities. There are far more of them than there needs to be. The abundance of water utilities impedes planning, capital raising, and worst of all, hinders providing the safest water possible for the nearly 300 million Americans who rely on these entities for their household water.

Nationwide today there are 51,535 drinking water utilities, or about, on average, more than 16 of them for every county in the U.S. If someone were designing a system of water utilities today, no responsible person or committee seeking efficiency, cost controls, and high-quality drinking water would conclude that having thousands of them—let alone tens of thousands—makes any sense. If progress is going to be made in rethinking drinking water in the U.S., the first step that should be taken would be to bring about a broad consolidation of America's water utilities.

The explosive growth in these entities is tied, in part, to the existence of many small communities in a very large country, many of whom want to have authority over something as important to their destiny as their drinking water. In addition, especially from the end of World War II and the postwar economic boom until the early 1970s, real estate developers used cheaper land and lower taxes to build new communities near, but not in, urban centers. For reasons of identity, cost savings, and control, the developers and the communities they created often preferred to have a water utility of their own, rather than tapping into a larger nearby system.[1]

This patchwork, decades-long trend of urban and suburban development has resulted in many very small water utilities. As shown on the chart "Water Utilities and Whom They Serve" below, more than half of the 51,535 water utilities in the U.S. provide water to communities of 500 people or fewer. A trailer park with even fifteen year-round homes can qualify as what is technically called a "community water system," but which we refer to as a water utility. Another quarter of all U.S. water utilities provide drinking water for communities of 3,300 people or fewer. If you were to expand the list to utilities in communities with up to 10,000 people, an additional 10 percent of drinking water providers would be included. Thus, 92 percent of U.S. water utilities (47,258 utilities) cover small to very small—and often poor—communities. In contrast, just 426 water utilities provide water to cities of 100,000 or more. (The other 7 percent of water utilities serve communities of 10,000 to 99,000 people.)[2]

To make the contrast yet starker, 137 million Americans live in cit-

U.S. Water Utilities

System Service Population	Very Small 500 or Less	Small 501 – 3,300	Medium 3,301 – 10,000	Large 10,001 – 100,000	Very Large More Than 100,000	Total
Number of Systems	28,595	13,727	4,936	3,851	426	51,535
Percent of Total Systems	55	27	10	7	0.8	100
Service Population	4,738,080	19,688,745	28,758,366	109,769,304	137,250,793	300,205,288
Percent of Total Population	1.6	6.6	10	37	45.7	100
People per System	166	1,434	5,826	28,504	322,185	5,825

Source: USEPA 2015, as cited in 2015 State of the Water Industry, AWWA

ies of 100,000 or more. They are serviced by under one percent of water utilities. But in those communities of 10,000 or smaller, representing that 92 percent of the water utilities, a bit more than 53 million Americans make their homes.[3] Those 53 million people are serviced by 100 times as many water utilities as are the 137 million.

The multiplicity of water utilities and the implicit wastefulness of having so many of them isn't the main problem. It is that, for the most part, the small water utilities can't do what larger ones can. While small communities may believe that they have excellently managed drinking water services, the odds work against them—and those odds are getting longer.

Felicia Marcus is the chairperson of California's State Water Resources Control Board. She has become a national figure because of her leadership on California's drought issues, but her job is multifaceted, and it includes oversight of her state's water utilities. California has nearly 7,500 drinking water utilities, two and a half times the number that the entire U.S. had in 1900, at a time when the national population across a vast land surface was about 75 percent larger than California's today.[4] Los Angeles County alone has more than two hundred water utilities.[5] As is true for the U.S. at large, the vast majority of California's water utilities serve very small populations. "Bigger isn't always better," Marcus says about the size of water utilities generally, "but less fragmented always is better."

Among the reasons she cites for which is better, the economies of scale of small utilities compared to large ones is first. "With a much larger customer base," Marcus says, "you can do so much more. You can pay for new infrastructure. You can adjust to regulatory changes. You can hire specialized staff. You can buy machinery and technology you need. These small water agencies are managing on spit and baling wire. They have no cushion for a natural disaster. It is hard for them to attract experts to serve on their boards. They rarely build up a reserve fund to help them through the inevitable hard times."[6]

Mike Keegan of the National Rural Water Association (NRWA)

strongly disagrees. His organization has 31,000 water utilities as members, nearly all of them serving populations of ten thousand and under. He has a passionate reaction to the argument that people in the communities the NRWA's members serve have poorer quality water because they are serviced by smaller water utilities. "There is no correlation between size and safe water," Keegan says. "The issue is the quality of the governance and the sense of responsibility. If governance is good, the water will be safe. If governance is bad, the water will not be as safe. Flint and other urban utilities show that big can be bad. Water quality isn't affected by size."

Keegan points to the well-known aspects of life in small-town America, a style of living marked by caring for your neighbor and a spirit of volunteerism. Many of the small water utilities have part-time or volunteer water supervision, with sophisticated water management being handled on a communal basis. "If you have good quality source water," he says, "you don't need sophisticated treatment."[7]

While what Keegan says sounds logical, the numbers don't buttress his argument. In 2015, there were eighty thousand recorded violations of the Safe Drinking Water Act. Some of these were for something technical, like a failure to properly report or to test as frequently as required, and others were actual health-related violations. Since most of the violations require self-reporting, and since water utilities have an incentive to under-report violations, there is good reason to believe that the total number of actual violations may have been higher. But taking only the violations reported and cross-tabulating them by where the violation occurred, something deeply concerning is quickly evident: Water utilities serving five hundred people or fewer accounted for almost 70 percent of those eighty thousand violations, and a bit more than 50 percent of all health-based violations—even though these utilities serve only 4.7 million Americans.[8] Because health-based violations expose entire communities to excessively high levels of contaminants, millions of people were put in harm's way.[9] Reporting on these percentages, one study commented that Americans living in rural communities "could be at the greatest risk from some drinking water contaminants."[10]

To make matters worse for those living in small communities, the EPA has a system of providing exemptions from testing and waivers for fixing violations targeted at utilities servicing very small populations. These communities are not obliged to test for unregulated contaminants.[11] And even when regulated contaminant levels exceed the EPA's own safety guidelines, small communities can receive a hardship waiver that gives them years to get into compliance if they can demonstrate that they don't have the necessary financial capacity to reduce the elevated levels.[12] The idea behind this system is that, unlike larger systems for which such monitoring or compliance can be spread across many more homes and businesses paying for water services, small communities don't have the means to do so. The obvious risk, especially for the monitoring exemption, is that, as with Hoosick Falls, the presence of a contaminant isn't detected until after harm has occurred.

Even if Keegan were correct about there being no correlation between size and drinking water quality, demographic trends—both macro and micro—are working against his view of the world. They are also working against the people who live in the places that his organization serves.

It is common knowledge that, except for a few noteworthy exceptions mostly found adjacent to cities, population in small towns has been in decline for a few generations. Productivity growth from farm machinery has been responsible for the shrinking of agricultural communities, and young adults with opportunities elsewhere often leave their rural homes, returning only as visitors to places that are poorer and its inhabitants older. With existing water systems originally built on the assumption of a larger base of paying customers, the long-term macro trend of smaller, older, less well-off populations only suggests more trouble on the horizon for the drinking water (and otherwise) in these communities.[13]

The micro trend is equally problematic. There are approximately 300,000 water utility workers in the U.S.[14] They are, on average, more than four years older than the national median age (46.4 versus 42.4).[15] But those numbers are deceptive. Already retirements are plaguing water utilities nationwide, with reports of staffing vacancies of as much as 50 percent in some parts of the country.[16]

At the very moment that there is a need to be ready to rebuild the national water infrastructure and, possibly, to be prepared for the regulation of new contaminants, there is an aging, retiring, and diminished workforce in place to address these complex issues. With water professionals having their pick of places to work, it is likely that small communities with limited financial capacity will have an even harder time recruiting people with expertise as these communities make their way through essential changes afoot.

Water services can be best provided from a larger base. Hometown pride can be preserved in other ways. It should not hold back the essential consolidation of the bloated number of American drinking water utilities.

Keep Mayors Away from Water

Consolidation of utilities within a few districts of each state seems like an obvious solution to bring down the number of these small water utilities and, in so doing, to quickly build capacity. This approach would have several benefits. It would address financial issues by expanding the base of customers. The new, larger utility would be better able to attract and maintain a specialized skilled workforce. It would also give the larger entity the ability either to issue bonds or to arrange long-term bank financing for infrastructure projects. And, of course, consolidation would reduce redundancies. To offer just one example of many, the U.S. doesn't need 51,535 separate water utility accounts receivable departments. Whether run by public entities, private companies, or not-for-profit foundations, the quality and responsiveness of America's water utilities would only improve with a reorganization and consolidation.

As obvious as the solution may appear, it will be a hard sell politically. In testimony before Congress, Steve Fletcher, the president of the National Rural Water Association (and Mike Keegan's boss), stated his support for the concept of consolidation, but then implored the federal legislators not to adopt any solution to water problems that would compel such consolidation, even of utilities that are consistently cited for health-related drinking water violations.

"When communities believe consolidation will benefit them, they eagerly agree with these partnerships," Fletcher said. "However, if communities are coerced to consolidate, one can almost guarantee future controversy. We urge you to allow local governments the authority to choose when to merge, consolidate or enter into a partnership. . . . We would be very concerned if the federal government expanded its regulatory reach into this traditionally local governmental authority."[17]

Since a significant majority of federal and state legislators have several water utilities in their districts, change won't be easy. Water utility executives can be expected to lobby these elected officials for a continuation of autonomy (and the perquisites that come with the position), thus opposing consolidation. Without countervailing efforts by consumer groups and others to educate those served by small utilities, change will only come when the wolf is at the door. But waiting for an emergency to create this momentum will forgo an opportunity for a planned, orderly consolidation. Whether it is with carrots or sticks, or some combination of the two, it is good policy to urge and to facilitate the consolidation of the 51,535 drinking water utilities into a few hundred. Each state might have a separate water utility for each of a handful of regions.

As important as shrinking the number of water utilities would be to getting better governance and higher-quality water, it is not the only hard political sell. To improve decision making, the counterproductive connection between water utilities and municipal government needs to be decoupled.

Originally, the majority of water utilities were private, for-profit companies. It wasn't until the early twentieth century that public ownership of water utilities became the norm.[18] The reason for that new approach to governance wasn't necessarily to assure better quality water or service. Nor was it to protect the public from rapacious private water companies, because by the late 1800s, most private water companies weren't permitted to set water fees at will, but had to apply to a regulatory commission to obtain increases.[19] The real reason providing drinking water became a function of municipal-controlled water departments was because mayors wanted the steady cash flow that water fees could provide. Taxes would rise and fall with cycles of the economy, but water fees were steady and reliable.[20]

Over time, water services came to be seen as much a part of local government as public education, except, unlike kindergarten and the twelve years that follow, there is a charge of some kind for water. People came to accept that there would be water fees separate from municipal taxes. But, because water fees had the feel of municipal taxes, mayors often did what they could to keep them just high enough to meet current needs while keeping them as low as possible so as to not lose popularity with their constituents. As a consequence of this low pricing, larger infrastructure projects were kept on hold until a crisis loomed. Because cost containment became a priority, mayors and their water utilities became antagonists—or, at best, late-stage enthusiasts—of regulating contaminants in drinking water. Instead of embracing consumer protection, for the most part mayors were eager to save on the cost of detection and treatment at their local utility.

In de-linking water utilities from the mayor's office, utilities need not become private entities. The emphasis isn't on the ownership structure. Rather, what is essential is separating water utilities from the electoral sphere. In a reset of drinking water governance, the best structure would be for mayors to have no say on water charges or who runs the water utility. As long as mayors see themselves as standing up for the public in keeping water fees low, it will lead to them to make flawed choices in both the short and long term. In the short term, cost control will be elevated over quality control. And in the long term, deferred maintenance and needed infrastructure build-out will result in today's costs being levied on a future generation.

De-linking water utilities from mayoral politics, though, need not lead to unaccountablity. Just as the public rate commissions in the 1880s assured necessary funds for the ambitious build-out of the water mains in many leading cities, a similar citizens' council could be created with locals representing different interests. Ideally, this council would be filled with appointees with fixed, limited terms who are obliged to cycle off.

For those who say that it is impossible to shrink the number of utilities and to make them independent of a mayor or a city manager, an instructive example can be found in the United Kingdom. In 1970, the country of then 55 million people had one thousand separate water utilities, each tied to a local government. These utilities were highly segmented, with little regional or national coordination. Many had difficulty covering expenses.

In 1973, an important change was made. The British Parliament passed a water law that created ten regional water authorities, replacing all of the local water utilities. The same law mandated that adequate fees be charged to cover all needed services. In 1989, ten years after Margaret Thatcher was first elected as prime minister and during a period in which her government privatized many state-owned entities, the ten regional water authorities were converted to for-profit companies. Each was made independent of the local or regional government, and was formally freed from political interference.[21]

Today, there are a total of twenty-three water utilities providing drinking water for more than 67 million people.[22] Around the country, water bills have risen by a third or more, overcoming generations of underinvestment in drinking water infrastructure. In exchange for those higher fees, the drinking water system is more efficient and has up-to-date data collection and other technology. Most important, water quality is higher and the presence of contaminants in water is lower.[23]

Even if now entirely separated from local municipal government, the U.K. drinking water system is not entirely independent. Several government bodies play a supervisory or regulatory role. The water utilities' performance in providing high-quality drinking water is regulated, as are the price charged for water and the acceptable rate of return for investors in the water utilities. Another government monitor compares the performance of the twenty-three companies to ensure that each is delivering required services and also innovating their systems with improvements they can borrow from each other. Environmental agencies, which are independent of the twenty-three water utilities, test for contaminants in drinking water. Yet others check for adequate supply of drinking water and efforts at fixing infrastructure to keep future leaks to a minimum.[24]

Fewer water utilities. Better quality water. Ongoing spending on infrastructure. High-quality management. Mandated continuous improvement. All with ongoing government regulation and supervision. It's a model that works. If not exactly a fit for the needs of the U.S., the U.K. water utility system can be an inspiration for consolidation and taking politics out of water.

The Drinking Water Industry Powerhouse

The most powerful organization in the drinking water industry isn't one of 51,535 water utilities. With so many of them and with few having a significant geographic footprint, the voice of the industry has long been the American Water Works Association, or AWWA, as it is universally known. Among the AWWA's many roles, none is more important than in serving the industry's needs in shaping drinking water policy made—or not made—by Congress, the EPA, the Department of Homeland Security, and other federal departments and agencies.

Founded in 1881 in response to the rise of municipal water utilities, it first dealt with concerns like cholera, typhoid, and dysentery, which the then-emerging generation of new water utilities realized could be better addressed with a unified approach instead of each taking on these issues alone. The founding members sought to share information about techniques in fighting disease, but also offered each other ideas and approaches about business operations, equipment, and finances.

Today, the Denver-headquartered AWWA's roles go far beyond both its origins and its serving as the central address for key policy matters in drinking water. The organization is also a water policy think tank, a center of scientific research about drinking water, and a standards-setting institute that promotes uniformity in drinking water infrastructure, chemicals, and practices. Its journal publishes some of the most important articles for drinking water professionals.

While the AWWA's leadership proudly acknowledges its prominence in these drinking water activities, there is one label the organization rejects: drinking water industry trade association. In a strict legal sense, the organization is not a trade association. But whether or not the label is technically accurate, with its vast membership drawn from civil engineering firms, scientists, manufacturers, and four thousand U.S. water utilities, no other entity is its equal in reach and power in advocacy on drinking water issues.[25]

In rejecting the trade association designation, the AWWA's CEO David LaFrance says, "We are a not-for-profit, 501(c)(3), which means that we are focused on scientific interests and education. We are not a single-purpose advocate, and we are not a trade association. We educate utilities to manage for the public good." Perhaps what rankles the otherwise friendly and welcoming LaFrance is the implication that, as with what is expected of industry trade associations, the AWWA helps its members—here drinking water utilities—do what is in their economic interest, even if at the expense of a more aggressive public health approach.

Interviews with LaFrance and other AWWA executives make clear that the organization aspires to do what is best for public health. But that judgment can be clouded by the economic interests of utilities that do

not want to be burdened with the tasks that come with regulation of contaminants.[26] "We are constantly trying to balance protecting a natural
resource, costs, and public health," LaFrance says. "This is not an easy
task. People think that water is simple, but it is highly complicated. Balancing these three things is very hard."

When examples are raised about contaminants that might have been
regulated or regulated sooner, LaFrance says, "It does turn out sometimes that what has been done proves to not be great later. But what we
can say is that everything that we are doing is always in the best interests of the public at the time it is done."

Perhaps because of its size and prominence, drinking water advocates
often cite the AWWA as the reason for there not being more EPA action on contaminants in drinking water. For LaFrance, a lifelong water
professional, the concept of pursuing water entirely free of contaminants
is more fanciful than real. "The idea of an absolute standard of trying to
achieve purity of water is not as simple as it sounds. Utilities strive for
better, but there are complications." As such, he says, his organization
does what it can, but believes the best way to manage drinking water is
to follow "the process of balancing benefit and cost."[27]

G. Tracy Mehan III, a former head of the EPA's Office of Water who
now heads the government affairs work of the AWWA from its Washington, D.C., office, shares LaFrance's outlook. After taking pains to
make clear that all of his comments are personal and not necessarily those
of the organization where he works, Mehan says that when regulation of
a chemical compound is shown to be needed, it should be done. But he
says he doesn't believe utilities should have to incur significant costs to
satisfy unproven concerns or supposed health threats not backed up by
compelling data.

Mehan complains of a mentality of "contaminant du jour" in environmental circles, suggesting a trendiness in pointing a finger at an alleged
drinking water contaminant before moving on to make similar claims
against another identified toxic substance. All of this, he points out, is

an end run around the process created by Congress with the Safe Drinking Water Act. Although Mehan's work brings him into frequent contact with members of Congress as well as the EPA and other regulators, it seems clear that he doesn't use those interactions to urge them to do more to protect against these "trendy" contaminants.

Quoting the Swiss Renaissance scientist Paracelsus—"The dose makes the poison"—Mehan says that there are contaminants in everything. Those toxic substances, he says, are only a concern if good science proves that exposure at a certain level presents a risk. "Just because something is in the drinking water, doesn't mean you need to treat it. There are seventy thousand chemicals in commerce, and we regulate ninety of them. But it doesn't mean that any of those others are hazardous. We can't treat seventy thousand chemicals. It's beyond utopian."[28]

Leaders at environmental groups and others disagree. More contaminants should be regulated, they say, and, even if it is impossible to regulate thousands of chemicals, more could be done than is being done now. What stops that from happening, some of them say, is the AWWA. On the other hand, they argue, if the AWWA used its undeniable influence, more regulation would happen quickly.

"The AWWA has an outsized power," says Ronnie Levin, now at the Harvard School of Public Health after a long career at the EPA in water policy. "They have the ear of Congress and of the EPA. They stop or slow almost everything that would create new costs for utilities. The group does some very good things, and there is no doubt about that, but if they were able to use their power only for the public good, drinking water would be safer. They keep the EPA from doing more."

Mehan scoffs at the notion that the AWWA has that kind of control, saying that the EPA—an organization he knows well—simply follows the law under the Safe Drinking Water Act. "If people don't like that," he says, "they can change the law." But he then makes clear that he doesn't think that is necessary or wise. "If we want more government involvement, we can get it, but that comes with a lot of other things. The question is how much risk is actually risky? Are we seeking a quest for perfection? Or are we simply just looking for risk reduction?" He also suggests that the EPA's Office of Water could do well with a far larger appropriation from Congress, especially to gather data that would be useful in a timelier implementation of the law.

Costs to be incurred by water utilities don't seem to come into Mehan's analysis, at least not as his primary consideration. His opposition is based on philosophy. "I know there are a lot of people who want to have the European system where it's a reverse onus, and contaminants don't get into the water because you have the Precautionary Principle," he says, referring to the European requirement that manufacturers of new chemicals need to prove the compound won't cause harm before it can be sold. "But I don't think that is the American way. I think that we should have to show harm before you can knock out a chemical or an item in commerce. You need to have good science."

As to the AWWA's close interaction with the EPA's Office of Water, Mehan not only admits it, but points to it as a positive attribute. "One of the problems about some parts of the government is that you really need to have a mind-meld with the industry that you're regulating," he says. "You need to have some knowledge of the world you are administering. We help bring that knowledge to the EPA. Because of that, we have excellent collaborations on helping to achieve public health goals. Because of that, we can work through solutions, even when there are significant disagreements."

With it being more than twenty years since the last EPA regulation of a chemical, it may be because scientific proof is lacking. But it also isn't hard to imagine that the AWWA's significant institutional power is put to work in support of the goals of the many drinking water utilities seeking to keep costs down. Balancing those possibly competing interests, Greg Kail, the AWWA's communications director says, "We advocate for sound science that helps assure each dollar is spent in a way that best advances public health protection."[29]

$1 Trillion *Needed*

America's drinking water infrastructure was largely built during three great construction booms: the late nineteenth century, the 1920s, and the years following World War II. The metal pipes used in the creation of the water mains in each of these three eras were made of different materials and utilized different manufacturing techniques. While individual pipes sitting in certain kinds of soil may last far beyond their life expectancy, a large percentage of the pipes from each of these three periods are believed to be coming to the end of their useful life, and all at about the same time. Generally speaking, the pipes installed in the 1890s last for about 120 years; the pipes from the 1920s, for 100 years; and the post–World War II pipes for about 75 years.[30] With frequent repairs and the use of smart technology, the life of each can be extended, but not indefinitely. Pipes can be put on life support and a few more years can be stretched out of nearly all of them, but unlike some Roman aqueducts that have lasted millennia, these kinds of pipes are never immortal.

Aside from looking at the calendar, you know a pipe has reached the end of its useful life when it starts to break. Ideally, the section of the water main or other pipe is replaced the day before it has its first break because it is far more expensive and inconvenient to fix a broken water main—the pipe that carries the water from a central distribution point to homes and businesses—than it is to install a new one. But since no one seems to be able to predict with certainty when that pipe is about to breathe its last metaphorical breath and because water utilities try to defer the expense of pipe replacement, even well-intentioned guesses as to the best replacement date are often wrong, and pipes often don't get replaced in time.

Although new technologies can detect a water main break before great damage is done, and even predict that one is imminent, the software and devices are not in wide use.[31] Most breaks get reported only after flooding begins and a sinkhole has been created, thereby requiring expensive street repair. In all, more than two trillion gallons of already treated drinking water is lost each year to these water main breaks.[32] Given the cost of transporting and cleaning so much water—and the energy needed to do both—fixing drinking water infrastructure could save a significant amount. By one estimate, as much as $10.2 billion is lost each year from this lost water.[33] Reducing water losses from water main breaks would also significantly reduce the amount of carbon fuel used to transport that lost water.

In recent years, as mentioned earlier, there have been, on average, more than 240,000 water main breaks annually in the U.S.[34] Worse, the rate of these disruptions is accelerating. A 2018 study revealed that water main ruptures had risen 27 percent over the prior six years, a sign that ever more of these pipes need to be replaced.[35] There are about 1.1 million miles of water mains in the U.S. Not all of them need replacing today, but, with age generally a helpful predictor, the majority of them will need to be replaced soon. Delay in replacing failing pipes will result in more cost for emergency repairs and more inconvenience, and worst of all, the potential for compromised drinking water quality.

The possible price tag for replacement of the aged water mains and related infrastructure could be more than $1 trillion over the next twenty-five years.[36] Although others have proposed it might be done at a lower cost, whatever figure is correct, it is a very large amount. To pay for this new infrastructure, unless other means of financing it are found, most Americans could see their water fees rise, possibly as much as 300 percent.[37] In all, according to a 2001 industry report, the average household will need to contribute about $10,000 (not adjusted for inflation) toward the replacement cost, potentially more for those in smaller communities and those in cities with a declining population because there are fewer people available to defray the cost.[38] To add to the burden, few municipalities or water utilities have built a reserve fund for this day of reckoning, having long used a "spend-as-you-go" style of financial management.

While the cost of repair and replacement may seem staggering, when paid out over the seventy-five years or longer life, it is less so. Indeed, there is an argument to be made that it should be even higher. James Proctor, a senior executive at McWane, Inc., one of the oldest and largest water pipe manufacturers in the U.S., laments that mere replacement of the aged pipes is a lost opportunity. While he says he wouldn't rush to replace pipes that might still have many years of adequate use left in them, he urges every water utility to choose technological upgrades when the day comes to swap out the pipes that are now in the ground.

"Existing pipes are just pipes," Proctor says. "New water pipelines could come with wireless leak-detection systems, and also with water quality and water pressure monitoring systems, to alert utilities in real time when there is a problem. The quicker a utility can identify a leak or the possibility of one, the less water that is lost, but also the less energy that is consumed to treat and pump that lost water. The systems embedded in these pipes can also help to insure better water quality by detecting a problem long before anyone is put at risk." Despite it being a better product, Proctor admits that his company's salespeople are finding it hard to convince utilities, particularly small utilities, to adopt what he calls "smart pipes." People are accustomed to pipes just being something that sits in the ground, he notes. They haven't come to think of them as part of what he calls "a utility's problem-solving tool kit" yet.

"Utilities are conservative, prudent, and careful," Proctor says, "and properly so. No one wants to take a gamble on something new because the cost of failure can be very high. But many utilities don't actually know how much water they lose to leaks. Without understanding that, they don't know how much money they could save." This creates something of a catch-22 situation. "Utilities don't know what their real costs—in lost water and revenue—are so they can't measure how much better off they would be with pipes that help them manage better," he says.[39]

The $1 trillion estimate for replacement cost is only for drinking water pipes. It doesn't take into account likely expenses for replacing wastewater lines, and rebuilding drinking water and wastewater treatment plants, many of which are also in need of remodeling or replacement. Nor does that significant sum reflect the funds that will be required to develop desalination facilities in dry parts of the country near seacoasts, or the costs of detection and treatment of soon-to-be identified drinking water contaminants. Add to all of this the coming needs for other essential public infrastructure like bridges, roads, and airports. Yet, without compromising our way of life, and with the understanding that it can be deferred only for so long, there is no choice but for infrastructure to be replaced or repaired.

If cheap water has been seen as an entitlement, it is only so because of the generations before ours that dug the ditches, laid the pipes, and paid for what we have been using for free, even if on borrowed time. The water infrastructure we enjoy was a gift to us. But now, for our own use and for those generations after ours, we will need to pay it forward.

The Wildly Varied Cost of Drinking Water

Since it is a universal need and a basic government service, as a point of argument, it isn't clear why anyone is obliged to pay for their drinking water. Other than in rare cases, there's no direct charge for police or fire protection or nearly any other municipal service used by everyone. Even if someone has a burglary that requires a detective's visit or a fire that brings out a fire engine and a company of firefighters, there is almost never a fee assessed for that service.[40] More to the point, no one is charged for the water used to fight that fire, even though it traverses the identical pipes as the water that comes out of the tap in every home. So why should there be a charge for the water in the house when there is none for the same water from the fire hydrant?

Of course, if there were no water fees, usage of water would almost certainly rise and likely even more of it would be wasted. In addition, if there were no water fees, the quality of the system would drop or taxes would have to rise significantly because water can never actually be free.

Rain, when it falls, is free, but every other part of getting water to people's homes doesn't come without an outlay of funds. The price charged for water helps to defray the costs of capturing, cleaning, and transporting it as well as all of the planning and administration that goes into all of that. And since water usage can be measured, the idea of everyone paying for what they use grew along with the development of water meters. Still, the public isn't asked to pay tuition costs for their children to go to public schools, and that, too, is a measurable cost.

The practice of charging for water began as a legacy from the first water companies in the U.S. in the early 1800s. As previously noted, most of the nineteenth-century water providers were private companies, offering a valued service in places where well water was hard to access or had grown polluted. When municipalities began taking over the role of the private, for-profit operators, townspeople were accustomed to paying, so mayors and city councils continued to charge, something of special value given the excess revenue it provided that could be added to taxes to pay for civic services.

Today, about 85 percent of all U.S. water utilities are connected to municipal government. Regardless of ownership, though, there is no uniform price for drinking water in the U.S. Prices vary wildly, and many public water utilities charge far more than private ones. Even within the universe of public water utilities, there is no standard price or obvious logic to what is charged. Phoenix is a fast-growing city located in a desert. It might be expected to have a higher average water bill than, say, water-rich cities on either coast, such as Boston or San Francisco. But that isn't the case. Boston's average water bill is about 20 percent higher and San Francisco's nearly 40 percent more than in Phoenix.[41]

Even more remarkable, geography plays little part in water fees. Two adjoining communities in the same state getting water from the same source often pay significantly different water charges. In a startling example, in 2017 the *Chicago Tribune* had a fascinating three-part report on drinking water in Chicago and its suburbs. There were many important takeaways from these news stories, one of which was that few of the 163 Chicago-area towns whose water utilities got their water from Lake

Michigan priced the water the same. What made this pricing difference
so surprising was that not only did all of these water utilities get their
water from the same source, but all made use of the Chicago water utility to draw the water from the lake and to then clean it before pumping
it out to the surrounding towns. The differences weren't a few pennies;
comparing the most expensive to the least in these towns, the gap was
as much as 600 percent. Even more surprising, on average, the ten poorest of the 163 towns paid 31 percent more for their water than the ten
most affluent ones. And majority black towns, on average, paid more for
their drinking water than the average price paid by predominantly white
towns.[42]

While racial disparity and economic injustice would seem to jump
out from the report, other factors are also at play. Many of the majority
black and/or poor towns in this 163-town cohort have shrinking populations, causing those left behind to pay more to cover fixed overhead
costs. Likewise, these towns often have aged water mains that frequently
leak or break. This requires the towns to pay for lost water, which can
approach 40 percent of the total charges. But without adequate funds to
replace the failing infrastructure, these towns make the decision to let
the water mains go without repair or replacement, and to pass along the
cost of that lost water in their bills. And because each of these 163 towns
is independent of the other, the farther a town is from Chicago where
the water is sourced, as is appropriate, the higher the cost to transport
the water there. But that extra transportation cost doesn't account for
most of the highest water charges.

The worst of the reasons for higher water fees, especially in poor communities, is that water fees are a substitute for other sources of government revenue in places with low property taxes and little or no sales tax
or business tax receipts. Although labeled as water fees in these under-
resourced communities, the payments are only partially used for water.
Some or most of these mislabeled water fees (and sewage fees, too) are
often used as a cover for revenue generation by local governments.[43] If a

similar practice were being perpetrated by a business instead of a government, there would be demands for prosecution of what is a consumer fraud.

Despite the widely disparate prices for drinking water in the U.S. at large, water fees are still a mostly minuscule part of the family budget. Cell phone and internet service can be among a household's greatest expenses, and cable television charges have grown at more than double the rate of inflation since 2000.[44] A study that tracked household expenses in the U.S. found that electricity and telephone charges each consumed about 2.5 percent of household expenditures while water and sewage fees taken together (the study reported them as one) came to just one percent.[45] While that number is an average and doesn't reflect the burden of actual water fees on some poor communities, it does suggest that there may be some flexibility for most Americans to have water fees rise. If that does happen, the revenue generated from these increased fees should be used exclusively for water-related needs such as sourcing water, cleaning it, fixing infrastructure, hiring qualified staff, and running the utility as well as developing a reserve fund.

In microcosm, the 163 water utilities in the greater Chicago area stand as an example of what is wrong with America's drinking water industry. As seen here, there would be an immediate benefit from their being consolidated. Such a move would save on expenses and enhance expertise in reducing water losses. At the same time, the mayors of these 163 towns have shown what happens when having water utilities keeping water prices low is a higher priority than having those utilities run efficiently. Politics and water services don't mix. And finally, in these 163 towns with ever-greater volumes of water losses, that lost water is a foreshadowing of what will be happening across the U.S. if water mains don't begin to be replaced.

The current drinking water structure works against the public interest in each of these ways, but most especially in getting the best water possible for the water fees paid. Restructuring of America's water industry will create benefits for most Americans, bringing about more efficiency, cost savings, professionalization of the labor pool, and better quality drinking water.[46] Water fees will rise, and, generally, they should. But, it will be for better water and better service, both of which are more logical reasons than paying extra for needlessly lost water. The only ones likely to be disappointed by a restructuring of America's drinking water industry will be the tens of thousands of redundant board members and executives at the water utilities that will be consolidated.

PART III

SOLUTIONS

Eight

PUSHING THE EPA TO DO MORE

"Can you imagine, if we made our societal decisions as if
the safety of drinking water mattered most of all?. . . .
This would lead to better drinking water,
fewer climate impacts, cleaner air, and a healthier nation."
—Lynn Thorp,
National Campaigns Director, Clean Water Action

WHEN THE WORDS "clean water" are used by people who care about the environment, they aren't usually talking about what comes out of the tap in your home. In the environmental world, clean water efforts are more apt to be concerned with protecting lakes and rivers. And while it is important work to safeguard America's waterways from ongoing assault, more people, more organizations, and more money are needed to accelerate efforts in safe drinking water.

Because fewer donations go to drinking water efforts, there is a shortage of talented staff available to educate elected officials, to lobby for new legislation, or to coordinate with federal and state agencies in the drafting of new regulations. Likewise, the funding gap results in far less independent scientific research being conducted on the effects of contaminants in drinking water. Without organizations to sponsor it, there are fewer think tanks offering public policy solutions for, among other problems, how to fix governance, infrastructure, and aging manpower at water utilities. The direct effect of this deficit—financial, institutional, and intellectual—is straightforward: lower quality drinking water for millions of Americans.

To be sure, there are many local organizations focused on specific drinking water needs. But few of them have the necessary support to do much more than scrape along. In any event, they are rarely a match against the well-funded and better-organized chemical companies and drinking water utilities that often oppose their initiatives. These small, local groups would do well to form a national clearinghouse parent organization to provide ideas and to help share best practices as well as to assist in fundraising.

Within the national environmental groups, a few people and organizations stand out as examples for their efforts in improving the safety of drinking water. Even if much more is needed, the life work of the individuals—and the groups that provide a platform for their activities—may inspire others to step forward and to add more as donors and as doers.

"Have You Spoken with Erik About This?"

Like many high school students in the early 1970s, the fifteen-year-old Erik Olson often found himself thinking environmental thoughts. He had been horrified by seeing large numbers of fish washing up on Lake Michigan's beaches, and engrossed by media coverage of toxic spills and deliberate chemical dumping. Even earlier, as a young child, seeing his mother wipe away the daily accumulation of soot in their home from trash incinerators and coal-burning furnaces located in nearby apartment buildings, he'd often wonder what the polluted air was doing to the lungs and health of everyone in his Chicago neighborhood.

That young Erik grew to be the most important person outside of government in the decades-long effort to promote safer drinking water.

While there are others who have also devoted all or part of their working lives to the issue, no one has achieved a similar degree of influence or—at least within the drinking water community—fame. At some point in the conversation, a large number of the people interviewed for this book asked, "Have you spoken with Erik about this?" The question reflects both the high esteem in which he is held and the implicit understanding that the use of his first name alone would be enough to identify him. Perhaps that is also so, at least, in part, because, although the environmental field is large, the drinking water subset of it is surprisingly small.

Despite the essential and ever-present nature of drinking water in every American's life, it is a curiosity that there are so few national not-for-profit organizations working on this issue. One leader at a respected environmental group that has done important work in drinking water quality confessed that environmental activism follows where the funding is. "The relatively brief interest in Flint aside," she says, referencing the 2015 leaded pipes fiasco, "donor interest in clean drinking water peaked more than twenty years ago. The last time foundations and big donors were asking for projects around drinking water was during the fierce arguments over what ended up being the 1996 Amendments to the Safe Drinking Water Act. It's hard to explain why this is so, but it is a daily reality." She then added, "For many donors who want to give to drinking water projects in America, it isn't for quality itself, but for environmental justice. It's to assure access to safe water by people of color and poor communities." Her comments, limited to America's drinking water, exclude the large amounts raised for the important humanitarian efforts in the developing world for safe drinking water there.

Regardless of where the money gets used, the three main sources of funding for the environmental movement are foundations, very wealthy individuals, and a mass of usually smaller donations that come in from charity dinners and direct mail campaigns. Depending on the organization's work, government grants can also be used for some projects. But fair or not, several environmental organization leaders decry that the

dollars tend to follow the headlines; what environmentally-minded donors want to fund are mostly what they learn about in the media.

Making the problem worse, unless it is a story involving gross contamination or fatalities, drinking water rarely makes the news. It is one
of the reasons why not-for-profit organizations working in drinking water
quality in the U.S. were so appalled by Flint and, simultaneously, grate-
ful for the reporting on the story. Although the news coverage ended
too quickly to substantially alter the political landscape for drinking water
protection, the media reports, nonetheless, helped to shine a bright light
on the issue. It caused most Americans, donors among them, to ask if
their drinking water was safe and to start thinking about the consequences of contaminated drinking water.

Flint notwithstanding, the leading contemporary environmental news
story is, of course, about the challenges stemming from climate change.
Following the rule that what gets covered in the news also gets donors
activated, it is no surprise that fundraising connected to climate change
has generated billions of dollars from foundations, wealthy individuals,
and the general public.

"I won't let you use my name," the head of a well-regarded environmental group said, "but all of our pitches make mention of climate change
no matter how tangential it is to the project we want to see funded. If
we don't, we would never get the funding we need for drinking water
and other truly important projects. It's not a lie, just a bit of misdirec-
tion."

Failure to attract media interest isn't the only reason that improving
America's drinking water quality gets inadequate charitable funding. It
may also be a function of the difficulty donors have in figuring out which
philanthropic bucket to put it in. For many environmental supporters,
drinking water is more appropriately a part of public health, a separate
category in the not-for-profit universe. Paradoxically, for many supporters of public health, drinking water is seen as a better fit with environmental efforts. With neither group of funders adopting it as their own,

it sits as something of an orphan when donors begin looking for organizations and projects to which to give their money.

Wealthy people may also not feel the effect of contaminated water as they do with other environmental threats like, say, air pollution. For the most part, today's water contaminants are chemical compounds that may not kill or sicken you for many years, if ever. In the meantime, there are urgent causes crying out for immediate support—such as saving endangered species or preventing the clear-cutting of forests or fighting for climate change programs. The immediacy of these causes puts a more urgent claim on the generosity of many environmentally-inclined donors.

In addition, if wealthy environmental donors are concerned about the safety of the drinking water that they and their family consume, they can easily stock up on high-end bottled water or spend the several thousand dollars required to install a top-of-the-line reverse osmosis unit in their home. Put simply, wealthy people can insulate themselves from drinking water quality problems. By contrast, polluted air can't be controlled as easily with a family-by-family approach. Improving the air of the wealthy can only be achieved by improving it for all. Outcomes with drinking water can be localized.

Erik Olson believes that the total amount of donations earmarked for U.S. drinking water programs comes to no more than $2 million a year. "I'm not speaking about the money donated by the Gates Foundation or the fundraising to get safe drinking water for people in the developing world," he says. But Olson believes that ongoing donations of less than $25 million a year could lead to a complete overhaul of America's drinking water. While $25 million is, he concedes, a large number, it is small, he says, compared to the funds raised for many causes in the environmental and public health fields.

If it could be raised, Olson says that $10 to $15 million a year of that amount could fund all research and advocacy efforts, with much of it targeted at educational efforts for federal and state legislators and regulators. Another $5 to $10 million could be spent on the kind of targeted lab tests we might expect the EPA and state agencies to be doing, but aren't. "When there is testing that shows a local problem and locals raise the alarm," says Olson, "it quickly changes the politics. When people all over America realize that it isn't someone else's water that is the problem, that is when change will come."[1]

Filling a Gap in the Environmental World

It is hard to find a college or university in the U.S. today that doesn't offer courses in environmental studies, with most of them offering majors for undergraduates and many providing graduate degrees. The programs tend to fall into departments called Environmental Science or Environmental Studies, or sometimes something grander with words like Oceanic, Atmospheric, or even Planetary added to the name of the university department. It wasn't always this way.

"Until the 1990s," says Professor Jonathan Nichols, a researcher and teacher at Columbia University, "most of what we did in the area that we now call Environmental Studies or Environmental Science was tied to traditional earth science and geology courses with an emphasis on mining and extraction of resources, or civil engineering courses with specialized training for wastewater treatment, among other areas. Classes for students intending on a career in the environmental field got added gradually, and mostly beginning in the 1990s. The word 'Environmental' wasn't added to our department's name until many years after the environmental movement began in the 1970s."[2]

The growth in environmental courses has been a response, in large part, to the explosion of environmental laws and regulations. Companies now need to be sure to comply with an ever-expanding list of requirements. To do so, they hire in-house and outside lawyers and advisors to assist.[3] But as recently as 1970, across all U.S. high schools and colleges, there were only fifty-four programs in environmental studies.[4] Students in the 1970s and 1980s who were eager to take courses that would match all of the excitement around new environmental legislation and policy were mostly left to fend for themselves.

One such student was Erik Olson, who entered Columbia University in 1976 as a biochemistry major already eager to have a career working in the environmental arena, even if he wasn't sure exactly what he wanted to do. Halfway through his undergraduate education, he decided to take a break and reset. He took a year's leave and moved to his parents' home, then in northern Virginia, during which time he worked at the EPA in Washington.

Likely because of his top-tier educational training in biochemistry, Olson was assigned to work in pesticides. He soon made an important discovery, if not a scientific one. "I came to realize that people [in industry] were mostly unpersuaded by the science," he said in a recent interview. "People believed what they believed and the science rarely changed their opinion. But if those same people were sued, it would get their attention and often cause a very quick change in behavior." He returned to Columbia still determined to work in the environmental field, but now wanted to be a trial lawyer, even if one with a deep understanding of science.

Because Columbia University then had no major in environmental studies, Olson worked with a faculty advisor to develop a program tailored to his interests that blended relevant science and policy courses. Olson's customized approach to his education continued at the University of Virginia School of Law, which he attended after marrying a woman he met during his gap year at the EPA.[5]

Today, the law school at the University of Virginia has two professors teaching courses on environmental themes and an environmental law program that promises the students the "skills, tools and experience needed to make their mark as environmental leaders in government, business and the not-for-profit sector."[6] It also has an environmental law clinic in which students can work on real-world environmental matters. But when Olson entered the law school in 1981, there was none of that. Without even a single full-time faculty member in his area of interest,

Olson persuaded the dean to let him earn full law school credit by spending a semester at the National Wildlife Federation (NWF). He followed that by writing a lengthy law review article on the role of the Office of Management and Budget (OMB) in subverting the goals of the EPA.[7] Operating behind the scenes, Olson wrote, OMB wielded veto power over decisions made by the EPA whenever it concluded that an environmental regulation would be too costly for the federal budget or too much of a drag on the U.S. economy. Olson's understanding of the role of the OMB in blocking or limiting environmental regulations was something he would return to again in his professional career as an environmental litigator. In cases he later led or participated in, he highlighted the role of the OMB (which acted, at times, in collusion with other federal departments and agencies) in halting EPA efforts to regulate arsenic and perchlorate, among other drinking water contaminants.[8]

After graduating law school in 1984, Olson was eager to work as an environmental litigator at a national environmental organization, but there were no jobs to be had. Instead, he accepted a position at the EPA where, despite his age and general lack of experience, he was given permission to represent the agency in federal cases and litigate them, including matters involving drinking water. When a legal position opened at the NWF in 1986, he took it.

Soon after he started working at the NWF, he noted a gap in the environmental world and suggested to his boss that their group could fill it. "There were almost no people or other organizations working on drinking water," Olson recalls. "Cholera had long since stopped being a problem in the U.S., and with drinking water, you don't see or smell bacteria or arsenic or lead as you may with air pollution. People had stopped thinking about how their drinking water could harm them, even if there was still a lot of harm that could come from it."

Olson then persuaded the NWF to get involved and for the organization to serve as a counterweight to the efforts of industry and water utilities who were working to stop or slow the EPA's drinking water regulations. He also got the NWF to allow the still not-yet-thirty-year-old

Olson to play a leading role. With the debate surrounding what became the 1986 Amendments to the Safe Drinking Water Act then heating up in Congress, Olson also got a chance to have some input into the final version of the bill and, even more importantly, to develop deep insight into what the amendments required the EPA to do.

At this point, Olson made another important discovery, this one also not scientific: Just because a law is passed doesn't mean that it will be enforced. "The EPA drinking water office has mostly had a sleepy leadership filled with 'Get-Along-Gang' types," Olson says. "Without some outside force compelling them to do more [in drinking water], they never would do so." As such, after the 1986 Amendments got passed and the EPA didn't move to implement the new law, Olson sued the EPA to challenge some of the agency's rules, alleging that they were too weak and violated the law. He was also involved in other activities to compel the EPA to do what Congress had required of the federal environmental agency.

Aside from his work in court, Olson had another idea as to how the National Wildlife Federation could help raise awareness of drinking water issues, including what the law said and how inadequately it was being enforced. In what became a recurring tool for him, Olson proposed the creation of a comprehensive, deeply researched report that could be used to educate several key audiences, including interested consumers, current and potential donors, other environmental not-for-profits, media, and members of Congress and their staffs. He soon began work with his boss, Norm Dean, on the first of several NWF publications called *Danger on Tap* that, he hoped, would inspire action by the many constituencies who could influence drinking water regulation.[9]

For the next five years, Olson litigated several drinking water cases while also handling other matters at the NWF. At times, to preserve financial resources or to share areas of expertise, environmental groups would partner on elements of cases. Following the March 1989 *Exxon Valdez* oil spill, the NWF and other not-for-profit organizations began lawsuits in an attempt to get an environmental restoration of Alaska's

Prince William Sound and compensation for local fishermen affected by the environmental disaster. The NWF made Olson its lead in-house counsel in the litigation, which caused him to begin working closely with litigators and experts from the Natural Resources Defense Council, an organization universally called the NRDC.

A short while later, an NRDC lawyer who was also working on the Exxon matter asked Olson if he'd like to jump from the NWF to the NRDC. Even with all of the responsibility the NWF had given him, Olson says he didn't hesitate for a moment and told her yes on the spot.

"There was—and is—no environmental organization like the NRDC," he says. "The NRDC was filled with talented people tackling nearly every part of the environmental world. Everywhere you needed an expert, the NRDC had it." As a going-away present, and as a comment on Olson's centrality to the NWF's drinking water efforts, the NWF let its departing employee take all of the drinking water matters he had started with him to the NRDC.

From Well-Bred Gentlemen to "Responsible Militancy"

As with Erik Olson, Gus Speth was a young teenager when he first became interested in environmental matters. Each summer, his family would pack up and drive the two hundred miles from their home in Orangeburg in South Carolina to Lake Junaluska in North Carolina. In the summer of 1955, when he was thirteen, Speth's family arrived at their summer home to learn that a local leather tanner had dumped its chemical waste into the body of water. The contaminated discharge killed all of the fish and plants in the two-hundred-acre lake. Speth was crestfallen, but years before Rachel Carson's *Silent Spring,* Earth Day, or the rise of the environmental movement, there wasn't much he could do.

It wasn't as if there were no organizations concerned about rivers, lakes, fish, birds, and forests in 1955. There were, but they were con-

servation organizations like the Sierra Club (founded in 1892 to designate and protect national parks), the Audubon Society (founded in 1905
to preserve bird habitats), the National Wildlife Federation (founded in
1936 to educate the public about wildlife conservation and to establish
government agencies to protect fish and other wildlife), and many others
devoted to preservation of hunting and fishing areas.

Although the conservation organizations may have anticipated the
goals of most of the environmental groups that were born in the late 1960s
and early 1970s, they approached the world differently. In the main,
the leaders of these old-line organizations saw themselves as part of elite
society. The heads of the Sierra Club and the Audubon Society were
mostly well-bred gentlemen with no interest in getting into disputes
with others. Certainly they would prefer to avoid something as tawdry
as threats or litigation.

The newcomers did more than change the name from conservation
to environmentalism. With their different worldview born of the ferment of the 1960s, they came ready to rumble. Bridging the gentlemen's
club to the world of the activist, they were happy to cooperate when that
would yield their desired outcomes, but—in what they came to call "responsible militancy"—they were also prepared to file a lawsuit or orga-
nize a protest when they thought they could get a better result by doing
so.[10] While this new approach was true of the group of new environmental organizations generally, it was especially so in the case of the
NRDC.

In 1969, Speth was living in New Haven, Connecticut, as a third-year
law student at Yale. He came across a newspaper article about the NAACP
Legal Defense Fund, which litigated cases involving discrimination
against black Americans. Speth asked himself why there wasn't a public
interest law firm like that devoted to the environment. He shared his
thoughts with friends who, like him, were in their last year at Yale Law
School. But he went beyond musing about the idea. Although he was hoping to (and did) serve as a U.S. Supreme Court clerk for the year following law school—the most prestigious post-law-school job in the

profession——he pitched his idea to the Ford Foundation, based in New York. A meeting in New Haven followed in which Speth and his classmates asked the foundation to underwrite the creation of the environmental law firm they had been discussing.[11] As luck would have it, at the same time as Speth and his friends were seeking funds for this specialty litigation practice, a young lawyer named John Adams, then working as an assistant U.S. attorney in New York, was in discussions with the Ford Foundation about a similar concept.

Adams had worked as a volunteer in a case suing New York's largest electric utility to stop it from building a pump storage power-generating plant that would have resulted in defacing a celebrated mountain along the Hudson River. Building on that experience, a group of prominent New Yorkers decided to create an environmental public interest law firm. They asked Adams to be a part of it. When Adams went to the Ford Foundation to seek its financial support, the foundation said that they would be interested in helping, but, as a condition of its support, Adams would have to merge his efforts with those of Speth and his Yale Law School friends. Adams was made the head of the new organization that soon became the NRDC, and Gus Speth was put in charge of the organization's efforts in clean water, which was exclusively devoted to clean lakes and rivers.[12] Speth's NRDC efforts never included drinking water.[13]

Today we take for granted the work of public interest law firms, but in the early 1970s these not-for-profit organizations handling legal cases on social or political issues——but without the fee structure of a traditional law firm——were a rarity. When the NRDC applied for not-for-profit status so that it could accept tax-deductible donations, it was by no means certain that the IRS would grant the request. So new was this kind of entity that it wasn't clear at first if they should more appropriately be classified as a political organization, which would make it ineligible for designation as a not-for-profit.[14] But following a favorable IRS ruling, the NRDC was successfully launched in 1970. While the contribution of the NRDC is mostly and properly thought of as being in environmental work, its role in the widespread creation of public interest law firms in shaping legislation and public policy should also be acknowledged.

From the beginning, the NRDC had lawyers from among the best law schools in the U.S., pedigreed attorneys who could have had jobs at the highest-paying law firms had they chosen that path. In addition to those lawyers, the NRDC also hired scientists, economists, and public policy experts who were seen as being as central to the organization's mission as the lawyers. With this team, the NRDC built specialized groups that grew from an initial focus on surface water, air, and toxic chemicals to include wildlife, forests, climate change, and much else. Over time, drinking water also became a specialized area of interest.

In each of these areas, the NRDC followed a common model. "From our first day," says Adams, who stepped down as NRDC's head in 2006 but who remains on the organization's board, "we knew we wanted to do more than just file lawsuits and be about litigation. For sure, we were happy to bring actions against corporate polluters, and we brought more than a hundred of them in just our first few years, but that wasn't enough. We wanted to suggest new legislation and be at the table as it was drafted. We wanted to know as much or more about the law as anyone, and then to help educate members of Congress on why they should support it. Once laws passed, we wanted to be able to go to the EPA and to help them write regulations in support of the legislation. And then, if the EPA didn't write that regulation, or if they failed to enforce it once it got written, we were ready to bring actions in federal court to compel them to do so. We would often be working with the EPA on some matters and suing them on others, all at the same time." When asked if the NRDC is a shadow version of the EPA, Adams pauses to frame his answer, and then says, "When the EPA doesn't do what they are supposed to do, the NRDC and other environmental groups are ready to push them to do more."[15]

By opening its doors in 1970, the NRDC was born at the same time as the federal agency and the laws that still shape environmental policy. Indeed, the EPA was also established in 1970, and the Clean Air Act and the National Environmental Policy Act (which requires an environmental impact statement for any construction project using federal funds) were passed into law that year. The Clean Water Act became law in 1972, the Endangered Species Act in 1973, the Safe Drinking Water Act in 1974, the Toxic Substances Control Act (TSCA) and the Resource Conservation and Recovery Act (RCRA), which regulated disposal of hazardous waste and landfills, both passed in 1976, and the Comprehensive Environmental Response, Compensation, and Liability Act (CERCLA), also called the Superfund Law, passed in 1980.

In just ten years, the U.S. went from having no comprehensive legal infrastructure for the environment to one that touched every aspect of the nation's ecology, especially water. Still, even with all of that, someone would have to make sure that the laws were followed.

"We Got Creamed"

Olson's greatest victory for drinking water may be the one that, paradoxically, looks like safe drinking water's greatest loss. It's hard to take credit for a bad outcome by saying that it could have been so much worse, but in this case it would be a fair conclusion. Always calm in demeanor and not given to exaggeration or public displays of deep emotion, Olson nonetheless describes this chain of events as "the greatest threat to drinking water safety." The episode was what culminated in the 1996 reset of the 1986 Amendments to the Safe Drinking Water Act, taking away the strong mandates for action at the EPA and replacing them with an invitation, if not a mandate, for inaction.

Almost as soon as Olson arrived at the NRDC in 1991, he began hearing of efforts to reverse the 1986 Amendments, which had required an active role by the EPA in searching for drinking water contaminants. There was even talk of efforts to repeal the Safe Drinking Water Act itself. Many mayors and governors from both parties, as well as water utility executives, were unhappy with the cost of enforcing all of the new rules introduced by the 1986 Amendments. Congressmen and senators were hearing from these powerful constituents about the wasteful imposition of a shelf of new drinking water regulations. At the same time, the EPA was moving slowly in enforcing those amendments, so more bad news—at least from the perspective of the water utilities—seemed to be on its way once enforcement would begin.

It would be essential, Olson thought, to establish that drinking water regulations were key to protecting public health. In addition, Olson was eager to show that, not only were the 1986 Amendments not a burdensome, arbitrary bundle of requirements, but that they didn't go far enough. And while he was making efforts to safeguard existing regulations, Olson also wanted to demonstrate that spending on drinking water infrastructure had been starved of funds for so long that the aging pipes and treatment processes were themselves a threat to public health.

By the early 1990s, it appeared that Congress might respond to the anti-regulation agitation, and begin stripping drinking water protections. To create the policy framework explaining why this was a mistake, the NRDC released a lengthy report in 1993 that Olson had spent the prior two years researching and writing called *Think Before You Drink: The Failure of the Nation's Drinking Water System to Protect Public Health*. The report revealed that contamination of drinking water was widespread and that toxic and cancer-causing chemicals could often be found in water coming from the tap.

Olson's report came with a 3,500-page appendix that named each of the tens of thousands of water utilities that had violated drinking water laws. It also pointed out that, in the vast majority of cases, there had been no enforcement action by the EPA or the state in which the water utility was located to stop a repetition of the violations endangering the public. After laying out a comprehensive list of changes needed to improve the nation's drinking water—many of which could still be listed today, more than twenty-five years later—the report concluded that Congress needed to "strengthen the Safe Drinking Water Act and resist efforts to weaken this major public health law."[16]

But Olson's activities went beyond his thought leadership.[17] In 1994, he announced the creation of the Campaign for Safe and Affordable Drinking Water, a coalition of organizations that could lobby for strengthening water regulation. Not only did Olson want to have the support of those organizations' leaders for the valuable advice and influence they could provide, but with the NRDC then having only 170,000 members (it has two million today), Olson wanted to be able to make use of these disparate organizations to trigger a grassroots effort. He wanted to have millions of geographically dispersed Americans prepared to call or write their member of Congress to apply counter-pressure regarding drinking water safety.

The organization Olson created and chaired ended up comprising more than one hundred groups, reaching beyond the usual names in the environmental arena. Working with others, he recruited consumer rights and good government organizations as well as labor unions who were interested in encouraging the rebuilding of America's water infrastructure. Olson also brought in many public health advocacy groups, especially those with patients with vulnerable immune systems such as children, those receiving chemotherapy, and people diagnosed with HIV/AIDS.

Olson's great effort could not hold back the forces of electoral politics. The 1994 Contract with America and the Gingrich revolution that followed led to change in Washington, and the arrival of a large cadre of Republicans in Congress. They were determined to cut back on regulation, not only because of pressure from water utilities, but also driven by their "smaller government" philosophy. Those eager to see a reversal in drinking water regulation cleverly harnessed the ideology of the newcomers to their cause.

Looking back on the 1996 Amendments, which is still the controlling body of law on drinking water, Olson remains filled with bitterness and regret. "It was good that we held the line and stopped repeal," Olson said recently, "but we got creamed on setting new standards for contaminants, and not surprisingly, new contaminants aren't getting regulated. We got Congress to create a Consumer's Right to Know annual report so that people could get information on what is in their water, but industry has neutered it so that a consumer who tries to read the report has no idea what they are reading."

Despite his scorn for congressional opponents of stronger drinking water protections, Olson saves his greatest criticism for the EPA. "The '86 Amendments," he says, "required the EPA to take action. The '96 Amendments created many barriers in front of any EPA effort to set new drinking water standards, and those barriers urgently need to be removed. But the '96 Amendments still gave the EPA the flexibility to take action if it wanted to. Because it doesn't really want to, though, it doesn't." This, he says, explains the EPA's failure to adopt even a single new standard for a contaminant in over two decades.

Patience Rewarded

In classic murder mysteries, arsenic is often the killer's weapon of choice. Death would be fast, with no puddles of blood to clean up before the detectives arrived. But not all intake of arsenic leads to a rapid demise. In smaller but regular doses, it can also bring about a slower death. Arsenic is a confirmed cause of bladder, lung, and skin cancer, and it has also been linked to kidney and liver cancer as well as to birth defects and infertility.[18]

Arsenic is a naturally occurring toxic chemical element that can be found in surface water, but is more commonly discovered in groundwater. It is widely present in drinking water in several regions, and especially so in the West, Southwest, Midwest, and New England. Aside from this natural encounter with the chemical, manufacturers of pesticides had long made their product more effective by adding arsenic. Arsenic residue from pesticides would then often be washed into groundwater or surface water. Similarly, arsenic frequently leaches into the soil and groundwater from improperly sealed industrial waste dumps.[19]

In 1974, when the Safe Drinking Water Act was passed, Congress asked the EPA to determine a safe level for arsenic in drinking water. Using a standard established by the U.S. Public Health Service in 1942, the EPA soon set as an "interim" standard a threshold of 50 parts per billion, but gave itself no deadline on how long that "interim" status might last.[20] In the years that followed that EPA standard setting, evidence grew linking arsenic's presence in drinking water with a variety of cancers and other health conditions.[21] Those early scientific findings caused the EPA to begin investigating whether a lower arsenic threshold might be more protective of public health.

When Congress passed the 1986 Amendments, it mandated that the EPA complete its studies by 1989 and set a scientifically appropriate standard for arsenic.[22] In the meantime, the level would remain at 50 parts per billion. For whatever reason, 1989 came and went with no action taken by the EPA on a new arsenic standard. Even so, the expectation was that it was only a matter of time before the review would be completed.

For Olson, setting a lower standard for arsenic had long been a priority. "It's a pretty easy way to significantly improve public health," he says. "The problem wasn't the science, because that was clear. The problem was that some of the places with the highest levels of arsenic were also where the most powerful senators were from."

One such senator was New Mexico's Pete Domenici, who had begun his political career on the Albuquerque City Council and, thus, was familiar with the operations and infrastructure in his native city. The utility there said that it would cost $200 million to be able to meet a lower standard for arsenic, an amount that would require a significant reallocation of municipal services.[23] Domenici, who, in any event, had been supportive of a rollback of the 1986 Amendments, was determined to protect Albuquerque's financial interests from what he saw as the imposition of financially ruinous regulations on New Mexico's largest city.

Undeterred by the evidence linking arsenic with a variety of negative health conditions, Domenici was prepared to significantly impair drinking water protection nationally in order to spare Albuquerque from supposedly massive costs—expenses that, the hype at the time notwithstanding, never needed to be incurred.[24] In September 1992, Domenici sponsored an amendment that passed in the U.S. Senate that would have put a partial moratorium on the implementation of EPA drinking water standards.[25] As it turned out, the Senate amendment generated a ferocious pushback from environmental groups that halted a vote in the House of Representatives preventing it from becoming law, but Domenici's effort and the support it received in the Senate was, as Olson remembers, gravely concerning.[26]

The arsenic problem was not limited to Albuquerque. In *Arsenic and Old Laws,* an NRDC report coauthored by Olson that got the inspiration for its title from *Arsenic and Old Lace,* a classic comedy about two elderly sisters who used arsenic to murder a succession of lonely bachelors, the NRDC reported that 56 million Americans in twenty-five states were drinking arsenic-contaminated water. Because of lax standards in reporting arsenic levels by water utilities, the report said that the number of those affected could be significantly higher than the reported amount.[27]

With the effort to roll back much of the 1986 Amendments gaining momentum, Olson was able to overcome efforts from the smaller, poorer water utilities that—because of perceived costs of implementation—wanted to see no further action on arsenic regulation. Possibly because antagonists assumed the EPA would never change the utility-friendly 50 parts per billion level, Olson and other supporters of stronger drinking water regulation were able to notch a win as the 1996 Amendments called on the EPA to propose a standard for arsenic by January 2000 and to finalize its work by no later than a year after that.

When the EPA failed to have an arsenic standard ready in January 2000 despite the then strong scientific evidence on its health risk, the NRDC filed a lawsuit against the EPA and also sued the White House Office of Management and Budget. Using some of the ideas first developed in his law school law review article, Olson argued that the EPA was being held back by the Clinton White House and OMB interference in violation of the law's requirement that the agency set a standard.[28] When a federal judge ruled that the OMB would have to disclose its records on the matter, the White House decided to quickly resolve the lawsuit.

"We had been making an argument to the EPA that the correct standard should have been three parts per billion, and could even have accepted five parts per billion," says Olson, "but we ended up accepting something else." In the closing days of the Clinton administration, Olson received a call from a senior EPA official telling him the EPA would announce that a decision had been made to drop the standard to 10 parts per billion. "He told me that he had pushed for five parts per billion but that the politics on setting it so low just didn't work," says Olson. "We could have proceeded with litigation and pressure, but with a new administration coming in, we decided to accept the proposed new standard." Still, an 80 percent drop was a success, even if not completely eliminating arsenic in drinking water as a public health threat, as Olson had hoped to achieve.

Aside from arsenic, there was another area of long-standing concern for Olson that was nearly upended by the 1996 Amendments. Olson had long been pursuing the stricter regulation of trihalomethanes, or THMs, a carcinogen that, as mentioned earlier, could be formed as a chemical reaction between the chlorine universally added to drinking water and organic material in the water. In drinking water parlance, these unexpected threats from chlorination are called disinfection by-products.

Initially regulated by the EPA in 1979, a standard was set for THMs at that time banning an *average* level of greater than 100 parts per billion for the combined total of four THMs. However, as scientific insight into THMs grew, it became clear that the level set by the EPA was not adequately protective against bladder cancer. As bad, it turned out, was using an average of THM readings in determining the amount of risk. THM levels are not uniformly distributed in water. Some parts of a water system often have far higher levels than others, and during warmer months levels can be much higher than when the water is cold.

Under the system established by the EPA in 1979 when it set the standard for THMs, a water utility would be in compliance if the THM levels across the water system over a year's time averaged out to 100. But consumers in some locations and during some times of the year could be put at high risk by drinking water with THM levels of 150 or even 200 parts per billion, even if over several samples the threshold could average down to 100 or less. The problem with the EPA approach became clear as researchers began finding links between spikes in THM readings and reproductive problems and birth defects.[29]

As with arsenic, Olson was able to persuade members of Congress on both sides of the 1996 debate to let the discussions on the regulation of THMs take their course, even if without a preconceived outcome. "Nearly every American was drinking water that had been chlorinated," Olson says, "which meant that, at current levels, they were at risk from THMs."

Even so, there was an argument being made to leave the THM regulations where they were. To counter that, Olson met with many members of Congress and also testified in Congress, noting that, "The risk of disinfection by-products was unacceptably high. What we have to do is to manage the risk by getting a balance between chlorination, on the one hand, which is still needed if we are to prevent an outbreak of diseases from bacteria and viruses, and, on the other hand, we have to lower [acceptable] levels of THMs."

Two years later, in 1998, Olson was rewarded for his patient approach. Following lengthy negotiations among water utilities, Olson, and the EPA, among others, the EPA lowered the level of acceptable THMs in drinking water to 80 parts per billion. Haloacetic acids, another disinfection by-product, also had a new level set of 60 parts per billion. But Olson and his allies kept pushing, and in a subsequent negotiation, the EPA agreed to tighten up the averaging provisions for THMs and haloacetic acids, effectively lowering the levels to approximately half of their previously stated thresholds.

Even with the wins in getting stricter regulation for arsenic and disinfection by-products, Olson still believes there is a long way to go. "It would be a mistake to think we are anywhere near where we need to be in getting drinking water to its proper level of safety," he says.[30]

Olson speaks often about the threat in tap water from Legionella bacteria, the cause of Legionnaire's disease, which is believed to have killed at least a dozen people in Michigan in 2015. He also frequently mentions protozoa called Cryptosporidium that killed sixty and sickened 400,000 people in Milwaukee in the 1990s, which he believes could return again in a massive outbreak.[31] Unlike bacteria and viruses, chlorine is ineffective against these protozoa. Newer technologies like ultraviolet light impulses, ozone treatment, and reverse osmosis filtration are all available and, Olson says, combined with better management of water pipes, could help protect us from both Legionella and Cryptosporidium.[32] But, he says, these techniques are too rarely used by drinking water utilities.

"Everything we need, we can do," Olson says, speaking of getting microorganisms, but also about lead, pharmaceutical residues, and other chemicals, out of drinking water. "We know how to do it, but we aren't."

"I'm Here to Make a Difference"

Ken Cook's interest in safe drinking water didn't start with a shocking episode involving a polluted lake or another environmental disaster. It started with a different traumatic event: the death of his father when he was a young boy.

Cook's mother thought it would be good for her fatherless son to spend his summers away from their St. Louis home on a farm owned by his uncle in southern Missouri. After several years of school vacations there, Cook learned about growing crops and farm life. As he was making college plans, his intention was to study agriculture at the University of Missouri, but the first Earth Day, in 1970, which coincided with the start of his academic life, aroused an awareness of environmental matters. Still attracted to agriculture, he merged these interests, finding not just his area of university studies, but also what turned out to be his life's work. His first job out of school was for the Congressional Research Service, where he wrote reports for members of Congress on agricultural subsidies and farm life.

After a few years there, he left the government to begin work as a freelancer, mostly with an emphasis on how federal farm policy could be molded to encourage better environmental practices. That led to a series of environment-and-agriculture-related jobs, but, as Cook tells it, he kept thinking about the broad use of pesticides on farms. In 1993, he started the Environmental Working Group (EWG), the not-for-profit organization he still heads, hoping to raise awareness of pesticides being consumed by humans, and to cause a change in environmental policy.

To aid him in his mission, Cook recruited Richard Wiles, an expert on pesticides, as his cofounder. Wiles helped bring EWG to prominence through a series of investigations on pesticides, the first of which examined the presence of those toxic chemicals in food eaten by children. Soon thereafter, EWG published a study of pesticides found in baby food.[33]

Looking for other ways in which humans were unintentionally ingesting these often dangerous pesticides, it occurred to Wiles that it might be worth looking at drinking water. Neither Cook's nor Wiles's intention then was for EWG to become a drinking water NGO. Initially, at least, drinking water was only one more lens through which to examine the presence and consequences of pesticide residues.

"We knew," says Cook, "that a variety of herbicides and pesticides were being applied to fields in advance of the spring planting. And we had reason to believe the water utilities in the affected areas were timing their testing for the EPA. Since testing was required by law to be done each quarter, in Q2 [April through June], the utilities knew to take samples either just before atrazine and other pesticides were applied, or as late in June as possible. In either case, the timing of the tests would avoid the spikes in exposure we suspected were happening, but the public didn't know about. That way, by design, the tests done by the utilities that had to be reported to the EPA wouldn't pick up the spike in the amount of pesticides [in the drinking water]." The intent of the utilities, Cook now believes, wasn't primarily to keep the public in the dark. Instead, it was to be able to provide the EPA with reports that would require no action to be taken to control the temporarily elevated levels each time pesticides were sprayed. The deception of the public was a consequence of the manipulated timing of the tests.

Wiles wanted to do something to highlight the gaming of the system. In early 1995, he helped to develop an initiative whereby EWG sent out a large number of testing kits, mostly to areas throughout the Midwest along the Ohio and Mississippi Rivers. Participants were asked to take drinking water from their tap during the weeks following the pesticide and herbicide spraying, and to send the samples directly to an independent laboratory.

When the results came in and were analyzed, the EWG issued what became a blockbuster research study titled *Weed Killers by the Glass*. The report stated that atrazine or one of eleven other pesticides or herbicides were found in twenty-eight of twenty-nine cities studied, including New Orleans, Indianapolis, Omaha, Kansas City, and Columbus. In about 60 percent of the cities, one or more pesticides or herbicides exceeded federal standards for drinking water, with one test coming back at 34 times the EPA's Lifetime Health Advisory level.[34] From this one small study, the failure of the EPA to get honest tests on drinking water was revealed, as was the health risk to millions of Americans.

Soon after completing the study, Cook and Wiles decided to expand the scope of the EWG to include drinking water. Through the organization's work in drinking water, Cook came to realize that very few people cared about water generally, but that everybody cared about their own water. "A report on contaminated drinking water in Florida or North Carolina," he says, "means almost nothing to someone in Chicago." But a report about contaminated water in Chicago would be of interest to almost everyone there.

With that insight, following the passage of the 1996 Amendments and then updated every few years since, EWG has embarked on one of the most ambitious consumer-oriented projects in drinking water. Using Freedom of Information Act requests, EWG was able to obtain drinking water data from every state in the U.S. After categorizing the information, the EWG invited consumers to go to the organization's website and to put in their ZIP Code. The EWG-compiled data would show which contaminants the local water utility had found in any ZIP Code in the country.

"We arc a relatively small organization," Cook says of the approximately sixty people and $12 million annual budget spread across areas of concern that now include drinking water, pesticides, and agricultural products as well as personal care and consumer products such as cosmetics and household cleaners. "Each time we issue a new ZIP Code database, we spend around $1 million. What is crazy is that this is a real burden for us, but that it is budget dust for the federal government. They could do it, but they don't. We find out and share all of the data that the local utilities are obliged to collect, including material that they aren't required to disclose on consumer reporting forms." Cook adds, "What we don't report on, but which I wish we could, is what other contaminants are in the local drinking water. With thousands of chemicals and not one new one regulated in more than twenty years, we can only imagine what health threats are being introduced from our drinking water."

Cook is a natural communicator, and one who takes pride in the impact his organization can make with "scientifically accurate," even if provocative, reports. But every study has to have a larger purpose. "I'm not here to produce laboratory research for its own sake, like a university. I'm here to arouse people, to educate people, and to make a difference," he says. But he acknowledges the long-term frustration of attempting to improve America's drinking water, and also explains why few of the large national environmental groups work in the area.

"The reason that not-for-profits don't want to be involved in drinking water," Cook says, "is because the Safe Drinking Water Act leads you into long dead ends. There is no resolution over long periods of time. There hasn't been even one regulated contaminant in so many years. It's disheartening. We are up against a system that's broken, a system where the public interest is opposed by mayors, utilities, and, of course, the many industries that pollute our tap water. And because of this brick wall and because there are other targets out there, and because organizations want to be able to show results, they go after those other opportunities instead."[35]

The Need for an "Awakened Citizenry"

Social media has changed the way that not-for-profit organizations interact with their supporters. But for impact, there is still no equal to the personal touch of a visit and a continuing in-person relationship. With that idea in mind, Clean Water Action, a drinking water and environmental advocacy group, has built an organization with two parallel strategies. In Washington, D.C., and in fourteen state offices, Clean Water Action works with government officials on a wide range of environmental and health issues. At the same time, in its state offices and with a small army of door-to-door canvassers, the group works to expand the number of educated citizens for whom cleaner source water and safe drinking water are a priority. Those canvassers help to develop thousands of new safe-drinking-water activists every year. Many of these people become donors, but more importantly, they can make their views known to their elected officials.

Clean Water Action was founded in 1972 by David Zwick, who, by all accounts, was a fascinating and dynamic person. A graduate of the Coast Guard Academy, he served tours in Vietnam and, like many at that time, came home disillusioned. In 1967, he enrolled in a joint program at Harvard Law School and Harvard's Kennedy School of Government, and while juggling courses at both schools, took a job in Washington working for consumer advocate Ralph Nader. Soon after he joined Nader's staff, Zwick decided he wanted to raise awareness of water contamination, and, as part of his work for Nader, he researched and cowrote

the 1971 bestseller *Water Wasteland,* a description of the challenges facing America's drinking water sources.[36] A year before his 1973 double
graduation at Harvard, while still commuting from Boston, Zwick started
the Washington-based Clean Water Action, where he would stay until
2008. He died in 2018.

Zwick had a philosophical impulse that guided his organizational
work. His grassroots efforts came about because, he wrote, "an awak-
ened local citizenry will always be needed to support the tough stands
officials will have to take to get the water clean." That one additional call
or letter from a constituent can sometimes be what tips a member of
Congress into either learning more about an issue or becoming a sup-
porter of a key piece of legislation.

Passing legislation was important, but only the beginning for Zwick.
As one current senior Clean Water Action executive tutored by Zwick
puts it, "At most environmental organizations, they consider it a win
when they get legislation passed. We consider it a win when we build a
new relationship with someone who can be an advocate for better water
policy."[37] Although he was a dreamer, Zwick was pragmatic in his approach. Laws oriented to the needs of the public, he believed, were rarely
enforced without ongoing pressure from that public. Corporate interests, he said, would always be well organized and figure out ways to go
around laws and regulations if no one was there to stop them.[38]

Today, the state offices of Clean Water Action do more than alert
people to call their member of Congress. In one of many examples, Clean
Water Action has a program in the greater Boston area that works with
communities to get lead pipes removed. Heading that effort is twenty-
three-year-old Maureo Fernández y Mora, who began working for
Clean Water Action as a part-time, door-to-door canvasser while a senior at Smith College. Today, working for Clean Water Action in New
England, with the title Drinking Water Advocate, Fernández y Mora
knocks on other doors, those of City Hall officials.

"We think of ourselves as community partners," Fernández y Mora
says. "We want the towns and cities to want to work with us. But that is

not to say that if they don't, that we are going to go away." In the aftermath of Flint, Fernández y Mora explains, city officials are especially nervous about the possibility of protests or newspaper articles reporting on failing to address lead pipe problems. "Most of the time, officials want to be responsive, but don't know how. It is a failure of imagination, and not of will. It is my job to show them that it can be done, and how to do it."

For Fernández y Mora, transgender and using the "they" pronoun, this is a moral issue. "It is immoral to force people—or even to allow people—to drink leaded water because these often low-income people can't afford to replace their pipes," they say. "The argument that the lead service lines are private property is mostly an excuse for inaction. If the municipality wants to find a way to do it, it will get done. I help city officials to figure out how to get there."[39]

Another example of the work of Clean Water Action is found on the other side of the country in the Central Valley of California, an area that includes the fertile San Joaquin and Salinas Valleys where more than 250,000 people live.[40] Most of the water used there goes for agriculture, and as a result of that, extreme problems in drinking water—nearly all of it sourced from groundwater—have been created.

The nitrogen used in fertilizer on area farms gets into the local groundwater causing a range of health problems, often making the water unfit for drinking for the largely Latino population there.[41] Yet worse, the pumping of groundwater used to irrigate those fields faster than rain can replenish the underground water supplies has resulted in the nearly universal presence of arsenic, something common when groundwater is extracted at lower depths. Clean Water Action's local staff coordinates with other local NGOs, and with state and county government agencies, to get funding to clean the water of nitrates and arsenic, and to develop new sources of drinking water.[42]

Back in the Washington, D.C., headquarters, Lynn Thorp, Clean Water Action's head of national campaigns, frequently drops the organization's catchphrase, "Putting drinking water first," into comments and examples. She was recruited in 1999 by the organization's founder, David

Zwick, someone she remembers warmly as a mentor and a friend. She offers what might be an impossible standard, but still a worthy aspiration that motivates her in her work.

"Can you imagine," Thorp asks, "if we made our societal decisions as if the safety of drinking water mattered most of all? We would get different—and great—outcomes. If we really cared about it," she says with a strong emphasis on "really," then "we would approach it differently. This would lead to better drinking water, fewer climate impacts, cleaner air, and a healthier nation."[43]

Drinking Water and "Environmental Justice"

Not every drinking water not-for-profit organization has a large staff or a national footprint. In communities all across America, small organizations work to improve access to drinking water and the quality of the water that local people drink. While nearly all of these groups lack the fundraising skills, budgets, and large professional staffs who enjoy easy access to Capitol Hill and the EPA, these gaps may be made up for with special motivation: The people whose drinking water is at risk are often family members, neighbors, and friends.

One example of this is found far from Washington, D.C., on the reservation of the Crow Nation in Montana where John Doyle, a Crow tribe member, has lived since he was born. Long before he became involved professionally with drinking water, Doyle was a laborer and construction worker. To keep active in winter months when work was slow or non-existent, he would take long walks around and over the frozen Little Big Horn River, a waterway he knew well. The river was the center of life in the town where he lived, used for swimming and fishing in warm weather, and as a source of drinking water all year long.

On a winter walk in 1981, Doyle—then in his early 30s—saw a part of the river that should have been frozen solid that wasn't. Steam was rising from between ice patches. He immediately knew that something was wrong with the water. He went to the nearest office of the Bureau of Indian Affairs (BIA), and shared his concerns. "They were very polite," he says, "but they told me to come back after they could investigate."

Doyle repeatedly returned and, each time, he was told that they were looking into what was causing parts of the river to not freeze in winter. Six years passed and one day in the summer of 1987, Doyle became alarmed when each of the catfish he pulled out of the river had sores on their bodies. Frustrated by the lack of response by the BIA, he brought his hunch that there might be a leak in an upriver sewage lagoon to the Indian Health Service (IHS). Another six years of promises of investigation passed without action being taken.

Due to the failure of the BIA and IHS to address this threat to public health, in 1993, Doyle called upon a reporter for a local newspaper and shared his informed suspicion that raw sewage was getting into the Little Big Horn River. A front page news story quoting Doyle, including photographs of the sewage lagoon, followed.[44] "The BIA and IHS were very unhappy with me," Doyle says. "They didn't appreciate my embarrassing them."

Two things came out of the local news exposé. First, the BIA soon repaired a faulty vent line in the upriver sewage lagoon and stopped the raw sewage from seeping into the river. Second, Doyle—then already in his mid-40s—became involved in identifying and fixing drinking water problems on the Crow Nation Reservation.

Today, Doyle is one of three co-directors of the local water authority, and one of seven people on the Crow Environmental Health Steering Committee working on drinking water issues. In both of these roles, Doyle and everyone who serves alongside him does so as a volunteer. (Doyle hastens to add that, in addition to those in these two groups, there are yet other members of the tribe who provide valuable assistance.) They oversee water projects in the 1.2 million acres that comprise the Crow Nation Reservation for the 8,000 tribal members who live there. Doyle also mentions that relations with the BIA and IHS are now more cooperative and productive than they have ever been, also helping to improve local drinking water problems.

In addition to these volunteer jobs, Doyle's "day job" is also related to drinking water. Since 2013, he has been on the staff of Little Big Horn College. In that job, he investigates the quality of local well water, often finding an array of contaminants in what is a common source of local drinking water.

Due to several laws that restrict the ability of Native American tribes to levy taxes, paying for new drinking water infrastructure at Doyle's and other reservations is a struggle. With the benefit of grants received from time to time, these reservations slowly build out their water facilities. Following discovery of bacterial contamination and septic tank leaks getting into local water supplies, Doyle and his fellow Crow water volunteers recently obtained funding from several state and federal agencies to investigate the source of the contamination. In addition, they are now seeking other funding for a comprehensive solution that will result in a return of the Little Big Horn River to its natural state.

The people of the Crow Nation are economically stressed. As of 2015, about a third live below the federal poverty line, with 24% unemployment. Ninety-four percent of students on the reservation qualify for free or subsidized school lunches.[45] Drinking water is of such poor quality in much of the Crow Reservation that—despite the poverty leaving little money to spare for extras—five-gallon disposable water jugs are widely purchased for use in homes. As Doyle says, "This gets expensive very fast."

Other Native American reservations in Montana and elsewhere face similar problems of financial deprivation and poor drinking water. "Water is the most essential element for living, and we let it become contaminated," Doyle says. "And then we have to fix it."[46]

While John Doyle became a late-in-life water advocate, Michele Roberts traces her engagement to drinking water and what is widely known as environmental justice—the fair and equal treatment of all peoples' environmental needs regardless of race, income or national origin, among other classifications—to her second grade class in Wilmington, Delaware. In the weeks following the assassination of the Rev. Dr. Martin Luther King, Jr., the teacher told her class "not only to mourn," Roberts says, "but to make something of the tragedy." It was advice that Roberts never forgot, and which has played a large role in her career choice of serving others.

Roberts works at the Environmental Justice Health Alliance as a national co-coordinator where, she says, she gets to live the inspiring words of both Dr. King and her second-grade teacher. In that role, she addresses the intersection of race, poverty, and contaminated drinking water, among other environmental concerns. Where industrial facilities have been located in residential areas, Roberts says, it has often been in communities where people of color or poor people, or both, live. Over time, drinking water supplies frequently grew contaminated, and only those with no other housing choices—once because of race-based restrictive covenants or now because of poverty and other reasons—continued to live there.

The people served by Roberts and the communities within her organization are among the most politically powerless and physically vulnerable of all Americans. Roberts and the other activists who work with her attempt to improve the plight of those in approximately forty communities nationwide by helping them develop the capacity to demand—and get—healthier drinking water, cleaner air, and safer handling and disposal of industrial chemicals, all things that those in more affluent areas take for granted.

Roberts gives Baldwin Hills, California, a majority black—but relatively affluent—community as an example. "Why is it that you can drill for oil in Baldwin Hills, but you can't in Beverly Hills?" Roberts asks. "It's because the people in Baldwin Hills aren't assumed to have the right to clean, safe drinking water, but the people in Beverly Hills are." When the permits for oil drilling in Baldwin Hills were issued, the residents there may not have known their rights, or, as a politically powerless community, may not have been able to assert those rights.

To assist those in the several dozen communities served by Roberts's organization, government agencies are encouraged to pass or enforce protective regulations for what may be these historically less-empowered citizens. When the government fails to do what is expected of them, Roberts and her colleagues assist in building capacity, which may include bringing lawsuits to compel the implementation of regulations. "We don't want special treatment for anyone," Roberts says. "We want everyone to have access to—and a right to—safe drinking water."[47]

Pristine Water Leads to Wide-Open Spaces

At least according to the stereotype, nothing is regulated enough and no drinking water is filtered enough to satisfy an environmentalist. But as regards the drinking water of five of America's largest cities, the opposite is the case. In these cities, environmentalists have been the chief advocates for *not* having drinking water filtered. Their reasoning is multifaceted, and goes beyond drinking water quality issues to a larger antidevelopment environmental agenda. Whether their approach results in the safest drinking water possible in any or all of those places is an open question.

In New York City, Boston, San Francisco, Seattle, and Portland (Oregon), or what might be called the Unfiltered Five, environmentalists have successfully argued against the application of the EPA's 1989 Surface Water Treatment Rule. That rule, which the EPA developed in the wake of the 1986 Amendments to the Safe Drinking Water Act, mandated that all surface water had to be filtered. But the strict rule came with an exception.[48]

If a city's drinking water utility could demonstrate that it had high quality standards and that the surface water that it was drawing from was a protected source, then the utility could apply for a Filtration Avoidance Determination. In practice, this meant that the surface water the municipality used for its drinking water had to be in a remote location and one where ongoing efforts were made to protect the source water from contamination.[49]

The five cities exempted from filtration rely on a claim that, because their source water is so carefully protected, there is no need for their water utilities to do much more than add a drop of chlorine. The reason that they don't want to be filtering their drinking water isn't a question of purity, but to save money. For example, in the case of New York City, it is cheaper to buy up land around the water source and to let it sit fallow than it would be to build and operate filtration systems. The cost, therefore, is lower on the front end (at the water source) than at the back end (through filtration), thus saving the cities from greater expense in providing drinking water.

Eric Goldstein is a lawyer at the NRDC who has worked closely with New York City in obtaining its Filtration Avoidance Determination. He estimates that if New York City hadn't been granted the waiver, it would have cost the city about $10 billion to build the filtration facility and then $100 million a year thereafter to operate it. While these are large sums, when measured against the more than 10 million people who rely on New York City's water each day and the forty-plus years a filtration plant would be in operation, it isn't as shockingly expensive as those numbers suggest. On a per-person basis, it actually comes to about two dollars a month for the plant and a dollar a month for the annual operations. But while Goldstein and the NRDC are happy for New Yorkers to save on these costs, their motivation isn't primarily financial.

"If filtration was demanded," he says, "then source water quality would inevitably decline. This would have implications for fish, birds, and wildlife in the protected area." Goldstein goes on to suggest that once source water didn't have to be protected, there would be pressure on New York City to allow farming, logging, and new home construction in the currently protected upstate New York Catskills and Delaware River areas from where New York City draws 90 percent of its water. "Once that happens," he says, "there would be a need for roads and stores and soon a move to bring in industry. Not only would the water quality become degraded, but the wide-open spaces that are now used for hiking and camping would be diminished or lost."[50]

Although not inevitable, it is hard to argue that the pristine areas of New York's Catskills and Delaware River—and by extension, the protected areas around the four other cities that have won filtration avoidance waivers—might not become more built up if the beneficiary city weren't holding back that development. While it isn't a certainty, without the need to protect New York City's drinking water, there could be pressure from local politicians and real estate developers to lessen or remove some of the restrictions. New York City would also have less motivation to continue holding the land.

While it is a gift for the environment to have these large unspoiled tracts, it also raises a philosophical, even moral, question. If existing purification techniques are available that make fallowing this land unnecessary, is it fair for what is, perhaps, America's most built-up city to hold back the economic growth of often poor upstate residents so as to preserve the city's drinking water quality?

But even if the conclusion is drawn that the tradeoff is fair to those north of New York City who bear the economic burden of this practice, it remains true that the 10 million people—New York City residents, tourists, and those living in several New York City suburbs—who draw their water each day from unfiltered upstate sources are still not getting the water quality that modern technology allows. The Catskills and Delaware River water sources aren't hermetically sealed, and, whether windblown or from groundwater or otherwise, contaminants do get into New York City's source water. Aside from some farms and homes in the watershed, there are also thirty-four wastewater treatment plants in the area from which all kinds of chemical contaminants may enter the water.[51]

While the source water of the Unfiltered Five may be cleaner than source water elsewhere—for argument's sake, it may even be the cleanest source water in America—it still doesn't address the presence of many unregulated contaminants in the water consumed by residents of those cities. People in New York and the other unfiltered cities are led to believe that their water is uncommonly pure or safe or tasty, but they aren't being given the full story. Even with the better source water, people in these five cities are still likely to have chemicals, pharmaceutical residues, and other inorganic contaminants in their tap water. If the EPA's regulated contaminant list actually reflected all of the potentially harmful chemicals found in drinking water, it is hard to imagine that any city or water utility would be permitted to bypass the filtration requirement.

When the topic of water arises, New Yorkers like to boast that they have the healthiest and best-tasting water in America. Tastiness may not be amenable to argument, but there is no question that New York City's water—and all of America's—could be purer.

It could even be as pure as the drinking water in Orange County, California, whose story follows.

Nine

WHY CAN'T WE ALL HAVE WATER LIKE ORANGE COUNTY?

"Water quality is a continuous pursuit. . . .
Since there are always new chemicals being invented . . .
we have to constantly be on the lookout for the next challenge."
—Mike Wehner
Assistant General Manager,
Orange County Water District

T HE FUTURE OF America's water may be found in the aptly named suburban California city of Fountain Valley. If drinking water is getting to us with contaminants still in it, the solution may not be to ban the contaminants, but, rather, to find ways of filtering the water to remove all of the toxic matter. Much of the source water that the Orange County Water District (OCWD), located in Fountain Valley, uses to provide drinking water comes to the OCWD even more contaminated than the water used by most utilities. But with years of effort, the visionary people at the OCWD have figured out how to make the final product—everyone's tap water—purer than the falling rain.

Because of growing water scarcity, Orange County was among the first in the U.S. to take most of its local sewage, put it through about as comprehensive a scrubbing as contemporary science and technology permit, and then reuse the water for drinking, agriculture, and everyday purposes.[1] Instead of sending that cleaned water directly to the tap—which it could—the utility deposits the purified water in the local aquifer. The water is then drawn out of the aquifer when needed and purified anew.

By reusing sewage, Orange County takes pressure off ever more precious freshwater resources, something of special value especially for anyone living in a dry place. Because of both erratic rainfall caused by climate change and growing population, reuse of water will become ever more common in much of the U.S. In every case, directly or otherwise, Orange County will serve as a model.

What makes what Orange County does so forward-looking is that water is cleaned appropriately to the water reality of the day. Most U.S. wastewater plants still treat sewage with a primary concern about what were the contaminants present before the explosive growth of chemicals in modern life. Orange County has reconceived water treatment to remove both the contaminants everyone else removes, but also existing chemical compounds that are found in America's drinking water—and new ones as they appear.[2] They don't wait for the EPA to designate a chemical as a regulated contaminant before removing it. As a result, by the time the wastewater treatment is completed, the water isn't just clean enough to drink, but as pure as drinking water found anywhere.

People opposed to reused water often suggest a more aggressive effort at capturing rain. Unfortunately, rain doesn't stay pure for long. Each rolling raindrop becomes a magnet for every pollutant that crosses its path, most especially exhaust residue from cars and trucks. Rainwater doesn't equal clean water.

Even more of a problem, there are enormous swings in average annual rainfall, making planning impossible. If you are relying on rain for your drinking water or agriculture, communities are certain to be either overwhelmed or disappointed. Rain is good as a backup source of water, but when you need water, you have to know it will be there.

A more reliable solution is necessary for any community that can't be certain that there will always be enough rain, or other water sources like a nearby lake or river. The most reliable of solutions comes from sewage—dirty water that, because of the 1972 Clean Water Act, needs to be cleaned anyway before being discharged into a lake, a river, or the sea.[3] Unlike other water resources that get used once and never again, sewage is a renewable resource.

Best of all, the volume of sewage is predictable. While the length of a person's shower may vary by a minute or two, it is pretty sure that they will take about the same number of showers every week. The volume of water used per minute rarely varies. Likewise, even if the total number of toilet flushes can be different by the day, it is a safe bet that there will be at least a few. The same is true for daily or weekly loads of laundry or dishes done. There may be small variations in the volume of water that goes down the several drains in a home, but the variance from week to week or from year to year will never be as wide as is with rainfall in any comparable period. The timing and production of sewage is certain and consistent. The volume of rain is not.

Even so, the impediments to using today's sewage as tomorrow's freshwater are obvious. The water has to be cleaned so that there can be no doubt as to its safety, and it must have a neutral taste, clear appearance, and no odor. Drinking treated sewage, with or without a stop in the aquifer, sounds disgusting to many, even if the objection isn't logical or consistent. Without a second thought, we sleep on sheets that others slept on in hotels and we use spoons that others used for their soup in restaurants. The sheets and spoons have been cleaned, and other people's sewage can be cleaned, too. Yet, despite assurances of the water's safety, once people know that the water being offered by their utility was recently in the toilets and showers of millions of neighbors, they gag first, and then rebel. The challenge is one of psychology and not of technology. It's called the "Yuck! Factor" for a reason.

Orange County's success in overcoming the "Yuck! Factor" objections suffered elsewhere in southern California is a leading reason why the county is water secure. But even with its world-leading water treatment systems, getting over that psychological hurdle to get the community's universal acceptance wasn't a certainty. The Orange County Water District had seen what happened when San Diego and Los Angeles tried to alleviate their dry conditions with recycled drinking water, and the officials in Orange County were determined to not suffer the same fate as their southern California neighbors.

"Toilet to Tap"

Municipal water departments are usually run by engineers seeking the best water outcome for the largest number of people at the lowest price. They aren't marketers and, because people tend to take their water's safety and availability for granted (and also don't want to see their water fees spent on advertising or PR campaigns), the officials who run the water utilities don't expend much effort on public education about water.

But as water grows scarcer, as more waterborne contaminants that need to be removed are found, and as consumers get smarter about what is in their water, communications and marketing at water utilities will become as central to good water governance as installing high-quality pumps and smart pipes. Whether the public is asking for it or not, water officials need to make sure that their customers know what is being done to make their water as clean as current technology allows. Communications will never be more than a very small amount of any water utility's budget, but it is a wise use of funds.

The need for ongoing public engagement and education by water utilities was vividly demonstrated short distances north and south of Orange County beginning in the 1980s when a few southern California cities decided to address growing scarcity. Going back to the 1930s, ever greater amounts of water used in southern California originated hundreds of miles away in the relatively water-abundant northern part of the state. The water had to be shipped to the more populous south, a

journey that required enormous expenditures of energy, and also significant expense to transport it.[4] Additional water came to southern California from out of state, primarily in the form of Colorado River water,
but that water was also in great demand by the more than two hundred
communities, and many more farms, that the river passed through before getting to southern California.[5]

Aquifers in southern California augmented the large volume of imported water. But the amount of groundwater being pumped out of those
local resources was being depleted far faster than the volume being added
back in by rain or otherwise. As such, officials responsible for providing
water to those growing southern California cities and towns could easily see a day of reckoning when this unsustainable practice of withdraw-
als exceeding deposits would disrupt their communities and economies.
With overtaxed aquifers and natural limits on the amount of water available from northern California and the Colorado River, adding treated
sewage to aquifers that fed municipal water supplies seemed like a logical way to augment the local water available.

Because consumers weren't properly prepared by their water authorities as to how this new recycling process would work and what safety
precautions were being taken, the concept of drinking what had been
sewage (regardless of how much the water had been cleaned) provoked
lots of opposition. This resistance movement became organized around
a three-word alliteration—"Toilet to Tap." The phrase was intended to
evoke revulsion and, with it, opposition. It succeeded in both.

Several people have been given credit for creating the Toilet to Tap
phrase. Its actual author, Dr. Forest Tennant, isn't some anti-government
gadfly or marketing whiz. He is a medical doctor who earned a PhD,
and even served in a part-time role as mayor of West Covina, about
twenty miles east of Los Angeles. When he wasn't doing mayoral work
on behalf of the 85,000 residents of his town, Tennant worked locally
in a public health office and taught graduate students at UCLA in health
policy and sanitation.

In the mid-1980s, Tennant learned that the water authority responsible for the two million people who lived in the San Gabriel Valley where West Covina was located was planning on reusing local sewage to augment the aquifer that provided much of the local drinking water. A lonely voice of opposition, he was convinced it had to be stopped.

"This was around the time when Hepatitis C and AIDS had come into popular consciousness," Tennant says. "The water authority hadn't shown that they could guarantee that those viruses wouldn't be transferred into the recycled water. Without being sure of that, they were putting the health of millions of people in danger."

Despite his certainty that, even with growing water scarcity, the recycling plan was filled with unnecessary risk, he failed to get others equally engaged. It looked like the plan would go through. Shortly before a final, likely irreversible, decision was to be made at a public water authority meeting, it occurred to Tennant that he needed to reframe the issue. In a flash, the phrase "Toilet to Tap" came to him. He was correct in his guess that speaking of it that way might help to get more people to express opposition. In the weeks that followed, using every spare moment he had, Tennant got signs made and used the new phrase again and again. People began to take notice.

What would have otherwise been sure to have been a sleepy water utility meeting ended up being well attended by alarmed citizens worried about their water. For good measure, several days before the hearing, Tennant scoured local junkyards and bought more than a hundred discarded porcelain toilet bowls. He lined the walkway into the hearing with them. Reflecting on his use of guerrilla and grassroots marketing, Tennant, now in his late seventies and running a palliative care and pain clinic in West Covina, says, "We made everyone walk through the toilets to remind them of where the water was coming from."[6]

With certainty that community opposition would now kill the project, the water authority accepted a compromise. The utility could use treated sewage for irrigating the local freeway's grassy embankments, which would save the freshwater then being used for that, but no treated sewage would be reused for human consumption.[7]

It would be more than ten years, in 1997, before another major effort would be made to take sewage and use it in a local aquifer. This time
the location was San Diego, California's second largest city. Nearly
90 percent of San Diego's water was then shipped from northern California or from the Colorado River, with very little local water on hand
for the fast-growing city.[8] The San Diego County Water Authority announced plans for the creation of the San Diego Water Re-Purification
Project, a euphemistic description of reusing treated sewage for drinking water.

By chance, the plan for San Diego's "Re-Purification" project got announced around the start of Sweeps Week, a period when television sta-
tions try to maximize viewership as local advertising prices get set for the
coming six months based upon ratings achieved during that measured
week. An enterprising veteran consumer affairs reporter at the ABC-TV
affiliate in San Diego, Marti Emerald, jumped all over the "Re-Purification"
story. She had learned of the Toilet to Tap revolt in West Covina from a
few local San Diego politicians she had interviewed for what became a
heavily promoted, five-part Sweeps Week consumer report.

Few San Diegans knew of the earlier episode, and the week-long news
series—promoted as "Toilet to Tap"—took on a shocking tone. Emerald had a toilet rigged up to a pipe connected to a kitchen sink, and used
that visual in all of the TV station's on-air promotion. In case anyone
missed the point, a female actor was shown drinking from the specially
constructed device, who then simulated vomiting. The "Special Report"
became a major topic of local conversation, and one amplified by the
clever, if manipulative, promotional spot as well as other media reporting on the public's reaction to it.

The Re-Purification Project quickly became toxic.[9] Politicians re-
sponding to the outraged public called for the program to be killed. It
was, but to make sure that it couldn't be resurrected, the San Diego City
Council passed an ordinance barring the use of any city employee or the
spending of any city funds on any project involving the reuse of treated
water for drinking purposes, whether such actions were directly or

indirectly involved with water production. No city official could reengage with "re-purified water" without being in violation of the ordinance.[10]

But there was more to come in the Toilet to Tap revolt. This time, the failure to reach out to the public came at a cost of tens of millions of dollars, many multiples of what a consumer education program would have cost.

In 1995, with little public discussion, the Los Angeles Department of Water and Power had begun planning for the local reuse of treated wastewater. A pipeline project, budgeted at $55 million, was authorized, and city water officials planned to transfer treated sewage from a municipal wastewater treatment plant via that pipe to an aquifer and from there to the public water supply.[11] By 2000, three years after the San Diego episode, the money had been spent and the pipeline was completed, but a citizens' revolt stopped the infrastructure project before it could go live. This time, the Toilet to Tap mantra was wielded by Gerald Silver, a college professor and the founder of a community watchdog group called Homeowners of Encino. Silver volunteered large amounts of his time challenging zoning activities that he thought violated the interests of the average person in Encino and surrounding areas.

When Los Angeles was ready to turn on the spigot taking treated sewage and piping it to an aquifer for later reuse in the drinking water supply of the city, Silver was experienced in asking questions of bureaucrats and city officials. When he thought appropriate, he used these skills to get projects delayed for more study—or, when necessary, canceled. He went to the meeting where final discussion was to be held on opening the pipe.

"It was a meeting of enormous consequence for the future of L.A.," he says, but one "attended by only eleven people, and no media." Silver objected to the project moving forward without more clarity on safety, but he was ignored. "They were talking about the science involved in the reuse of sewage as if it were all settled and that there was no possibility of harm," he says. "I wanted my objection to be heard."[12]

Matters took an unexpected turn after the meeting when Silver contacted a local newspaper to alert them to what was happening. The newspaper decided to cover the story, and the headline accompanying the news article included the words "Toilet to Tap," a phrase then largely unknown in Los Angeles.[13] Silver remembers that it "came to define the whole dispute."[14] And to devastating effect.

As luck would have it, Los Angeles was in the early stage of a campaign to replace a term-limited mayor when the article and headline appeared. Candidates attuned to voter sentiment picked up on the story, and saw Toilet to Tap as a smart way of getting media attention. One candidate with special authority adopted the cause.

James Hahn, then the city attorney, used the powers of his office to kill the already built and paid-for pipeline and reuse program. With that order, $55 million of Los Angeles taxpayers' money went down the drain. Although it isn't clear what role Hahn's order played in his later winning the election, after becoming mayor in 2001, Hahn instructed L.A.'s water utility to not reuse treated sewage for drinking water, regardless of purity.[15]

After San Gabriel Valley, San Diego, and Los Angeles, water authorities all over the country took notice of the southern California Toilet to Tap uprisings. If water was going to be reused, it would have to be managed and marketed differently. Fortunately, Orange County had what it thought was a better idea.

Seawater and Freshwater Don't Mix

Orange County got its name and independent status in 1889. The large agricultural district had been part of Los Angeles County when the discovery of silver in the Santa Ana Mountains in 1887 led to a spurt of migrants. State officials decided the area would do better apart—at least politically—from Los Angeles. Then, attempting to encourage others to come who would be wedded to the land, officials in the new county played down the get-rich-quick silver rush and emphasized the natural

bounty of the area. The name Orange County was chosen to evoke citrus groves, rich soil, and especially abundant water, even though the area
had recently endured a ruinous drought.

In the 1890 federal census, the first taken of Orange County, California, 13,589 inhabitants were recorded. In its first decades legally separated from Los Angeles, the district came to serve as a weekend retreat
for wealthy people in the nearby city—especially the stars and moguls
who built the new California film industry—who were attracted by the
same pleasant climate as L.A., but with wide-open spaces for farms and
vistas of grazing animals.

Orange County's population grew, but slowly. On the eve of World
War II, fifty years after achieving independent status, scarcely 130,000
people were living in the county's approximately 800 square miles, a population density of only about 160 people per square mile. But everything changed in the postwar years as returning GIs from all over the
country chose to build their homes and start businesses only a short ride
from Los Angeles. A cluster of high-tech start-ups and relocating aerospace companies helped to drive the local economy.

Tourism was also responsible for exposing large numbers of people
to the area. In 1950, Walt Disney began construction of Disneyland in
Anaheim, which opened five years later. The Knott family added attrac-
tions to their berry farm, and the plainly named Knott's Berry Farm also
became a popular tourist destination. By 1960, the county had grown
to more than 700,000 people, and the population more than doubled in
the ten years that followed. Today, Orange County is home to nearly 3.2
million and, if once sparsely settled, it is now, after San Francisco, the
state's most densely populated county.

All of these new residents and businesses were, of course, drawing
on existing water resources, but they weren't the only ones depleting
the water that flowed via the Santa Ana River and, even more so, from
groundwater found in local aquifers. Agriculture had long been a leading part of the economy in the county. As far back as the 1930s, farmers' need for water for citrus, avocados, and grazing animals had already

put a measurable strain on water supplies. During the war years, the open spaces and the proximity to the Pacific Ocean made Orange County a key military center, which also resulted in a large pull on water supplies.[16]

During World War II, far from Orange County, engineers developed huge pumps for use on America's naval vessels. Now, in peacetime, this same technology could be applied to extract enormous amounts of groundwater to assure that local crops and animals would have all of the water they could need. But without rainfall or other recharge equal to the amount of groundwater extracted, the water level in the aquifer continued to drop.

A small problem first detected in Orange County in the 1930s threatened to become a major one in the 1960s. Aquifer systems along the county's forty miles of coastline began to take on seawater. With ever greater and faster extraction of fresh groundwater from the aquifers, hydraulic pressure caused an ongoing rebalancing of the water at hand, drawing seawater into the aquifer to make up for the freshwater extracted.[17] That seawater came, of course, with a high salt and mineral content. Fresh and ocean waters began mixing. The salt content found in the freshwater aquifers noted as a concern in the 1930s began rising, rendering some wells unusable.[18] Unchecked, the salinization of the aquifers could, at some point, produce water too salty to use for agriculture or human consumption.

To address the saltwater intrusion, the county water authority could have taken one of three routes. First, they could have limited extraction until rainfall and other sources replenished the freshwater in the aquifer, but that would have had unwanted economic consequences. Second, they could have searched for new sources of freshwater, but alternative water sources from northern California, the Colorado River, and the Santa Ana River, among others, were already being tapped at or close to their limit, especially as many other communities were also in need of additional water. Or, third, they could have constructed a barrier to keep out the seawater.

In a sense, all three approaches ended up being used. Thanks to technology and conservation efforts, water use per person was reduced, even if the total number of people continued to grow. A new source of water was developed, even if not one imported from outside the county. And they decided to build a barrier to keep seawater from deeper penetration of the county's groundwater. Ultimately, the second and third options here—the development of new water and the construction of a seawater barrier—became linked.

Beginning in the 1970s, the county decided to take action on the seawater intrusion with a facility called Water Factory 21. Utilizing the laws of physics along with a blend of highly treated wastewater mixed with fresh water, county water officials hoped to push back the saltwater intrusion. Two miles inland from the Pacific Ocean, at a point where the seawater infiltration had already occurred, a deep well was constructed to extract salt water from the aquifer. The process of extracting that water created a depression in the aquifer and reversed the hydraulic pressure. To complement that process, two miles farther east, a second well was drilled, and the blend of purified sewage and fresh water was injected into it. As a result of the depression created in the first of those wells, the highly treated sewage was pulled toward the ocean, thereby creating a hydraulic barrier that would keep out new seawater from intruding farther inland.[19]

Because of the relatively small amounts of treated sewage utilized— initially, 10 million gallons a day—in such a large area and the high quality of the sewage purification, state environmental officials were confident that there would be no adverse health consequences.[20] Whether that was accurate required something of a leap of faith at the time, but the injection of purified wastewater mixed with some freshwater did what was intended. The mixing of salty water from the Pacific Ocean and fresh groundwater in the aquifer was significantly slowed, and unless over-pumping of the aquifer accelerated, the fresh groundwater in Orange County would be protected from further salinization.[21]

After five years of Water Factory 21 operations, the initial intuition of the county's water officials proved to be accurate. A 1982 Stanford

University engineering study reported, that "No evidence was found re-claimed municipal wastewater would pose a significant health risk," if it were used as a source of freshwater.[22]

If the injection of treated sewage began as a means of having adequate water to use to rebalance the intruding seawater, the safety of that re-claimed water opened the door to new thinking in the late 1990s about adding highly purified wastewater to the water supply. The steps taken by Orange County would lead to a transformation in the county's—and sooner or later, perhaps, everyone's—water future.

But before enormous amounts of treated sewage could be added to the natural freshwater supplies found in the aquifer's groundwater, more than just overcoming large engineering challenges was necessary. Mind-ful of what had happened nearby and in recent years, county officials decided to preempt a local Toilet to Tap revolt of the kind experienced elsewhere in southern California.

Killing the Toilet to Tap Scare

There's no documentation of who first realized that sewage could be re-used if only it could be purified, but likely it has been a yearning in drought-stricken and dry areas since before recorded history. As early as 1925, four years before the creation of the Orange County Water Dis-trict, local farmers and officials in Orange County raised the possibility of taking the county's sewage and using it to replenish the aquifer. The problem then and at all other times the topic was raised was the same one raised by Forest Tennant and Gerald Silver, which was the lack of certainty that the aquifer wouldn't be contaminated if the purification was less than perfect.[23] Aside from the risk of drinking contaminated water for any individual, it would put the future of the whole commu-nity in peril if the aquifer ended up unusable. It was a gamble too large to take.

That thinking began to change when the treated wastewater used by

Water Factory 21 was shown to have no ill effect on health. Now, by expanding the use of treated sewage beyond just what was needed to feed the hydraulic barrier, Orange County could have a perpetual source of old-new water able to keep pace with population growth and economic expansion in the county.

In 1999, water officials decided it was finally the right moment to draw up plans for the ultra-purification of the county's sewage and its reuse. A partnership was launched between the two halves of the local water equation, the Orange County Water District (responsible for managing the county's freshwater) and the Orange County Sanitation District (responsible for managing the treatment and disposal of the county's sewage). Jointly, they created a project called the Groundwater Replenishment System (GWRS).[24]

Still, as the project's partners began planning this enormous engineering endeavor with belief in its likely technical success, they also faced the same challenge as other southern California cities in gaining the acceptance of the public. As they saw elsewhere, elected officials could be easily frightened into withdrawing their support—even killing projects that had already been built and paid for—when popular sentiment turned against them.

To protect against this, the GWRS leaders decided to make public outreach as integral a part of the program as were the architectural renderings and the science underpinning the new program. "Even before we developed all of our engineering plans," says Mike Markus, the project manager for GWRS since its inception in 1999 and the general manager of the Orange County Water District since 2007, "we went to work on educating the community about why this was good for them and why it was important for the future. We wanted everyone to be enthusiastic about the replenishment system long before the system would be up and running."[25]

The water officials began with consumer research to get a better feel for the public's concerns. By this time, with Orange County located between Los Angeles and San Diego, a large part of the public had heard of Toilet to Tap protests elsewhere. Although most locals didn't know a lot about it, they knew that others had rejected water recycling programs. Without having more information, it seemed possible that people in Orange County could also reject the opportunity to drink other people's previously used water. There was no reason why Orange County residents should be immune to the "Yuck! Factor."

In addition, given how explosive reused water had become as an issue in other cities, it would be important to get every public official smart about the Groundwater Replenishment System. If public opposition became pronounced, politicians' abandonment of the project would be likely, but it would be important to have advocates for the system who could vouch for it before consumer grumbling grew into a prairie fire.

Understanding that there are many kinds of influencers, GWRS tried reaching as many of them as possible. Presentations were made to heads of a variety of community organizations about the new project, and why it would be good for Orange County and for each person living there. Open meetings were held so that the public could hear about what was being planned. Local media was brought in often to learn about each successive development in the project with the hope that they would cover the story and reinforce solidifying consumer sentiment. Polling was done on a regular basis to measure community attitudes, giving the Orange County Water District the opportunity to see what impact the painstaking educational efforts were having.

What may be most remarkable about this menu of activities—from polling to influencing elite opinion to grassroots engagement to media strategy and public relations—isn't that they were done, but that such ho-hum obvious and commonplace research and marketing were seen as path-breaking when done by Orange County. It would be hard to imagine a for-profit company of any size or an advocacy organization with a secure base of donors that doesn't do all of this and more. Orange County deserves to be applauded for these efforts, but it also is a reminder of how poorly most water utilities handle marketing, communications, and public relations, if they do anything at all.

Detailed designs for the seawater barrier and the aquifer replenishment were completed in 2002 when construction began. In 2008, the ambitious program was operational.

"By the time we opened the Groundwater Replenishment System," Markus says, "there was no opposition that we knew of. Everyone was on board." Even so, GWRS takes nothing for granted, continuing outreach and education to this day. "Broad-based citizens' support is as important to us today as ever," Markus says, "and we think of the media as an intrinsic part of that."[26]

The entire cost for the outreach effort from when it began in 2000 to when GWRS went live in 2008 was $1 million, or the equivalent of $125,000 per year. "It helped ensure the project could move forward and wouldn't later become"—as happened elsewhere—"a stranded asset," says Eleanor Torres, the director of public affairs at the Water District since 2008. "The first phase of the project was $481 million. Marketing came to just 0.21% of that."[27]

Because of enthusiastic public support, a GWRS expansion was authorized for an additional $142 million, which came online in 2015 and which increased the amount of highly treated wastewater from the initial 70 million gallons a day to 100 million gallons. A further expansion, budgeted at $135 million, is scheduled for 2022 which will bring the amount of treated sewage that can be injected into the aquifer and later reused as drinking water to as much as 130 million gallons a day.[28]

With the average American household using three hundred gallons of water a day for showers, toilet flushing, food preparation, dishwashers, laundry, and gardening, the new water that the Orange County Water District will be producing from treated sewage will be adequate to provide for the needs of the equivalent of over 400,000 homes and families.[29] This will take enormous pressure off of the freshwater demands in Orange County. Even adding in the amount of water that local farmers may consume for crops and livestock, it is clear that Orange County will soon enjoy near self-sufficiency in water.

What Orange County has done in engaging the public is the model for other cities and communities, whether in a dry place or not. Every water utility can and should educate its customers to turn them into partners.

Orange County's success has been a win for other dry places eager to make use of its most valuable renewable water resource. Years after Los Angeles and San Diego had rejected water reuse programs in the aftermath of Toilet to Tap campaigns, both—after seeing what had been achieved in public education in Orange County—successfully did the same, resulting in thriving local water reuse programs.

And in an odd postscript, both Dr. Forest Tennant, who coined the Toilet to Tap slogan, and Professor Gerald Silver, who led the upheaval resulting in the cancellation of the $55 million pipeline, later become supporters of treated wastewater being reused for drinking water.[30] Marti Emerald, the San Diego TV consumer affairs reporter who produced the five-part news story on Toilet to Tap, quit her job a few years later after thirty years as a journalist, ran for San Diego City Council, and won. While in office, she became an advocate for water recycling of the exact kind San Diego had earlier considered and rejected.[31]

Old Tools—and New—for Ultraclean Water

No matter how good Orange County had become at marketing and communications, there is no chance the people of the county would have allowed GWRS to spend more than half a billion dollars building the reused water program unless it could be demonstrated that the water was healthy and safe to drink.[32]

What is so special about the Orange Country purification system is that GWRS didn't require the invention of a new water technology or the use of any unique element. Every part of the purification process is also done somewhere else. The difference is that all of these different elements have been integrated, and then continually fine-tuned. This results in water that is as clean as water can be. No chemical contaminants—regulated by the EPA or not—survive the treatment process. Water that begins as sewage ends up being safer than drinking water elsewhere that starts in even pristine watersheds. As mentioned earlier, the standard used by most water utilities and water officials isn't to be as clean as Orange County demands of its finished water, but only to observe the minimum levels demanded by law. That may be clean enough, but not as pure as science and technology can deliver. Unlike other utilities, the Orange County Water District tests for contaminants that aren't regulated or under a current EPA contaminant monitoring program. The utility doesn't just try to bring levels of any regulated contaminant down to the maximum permitted level, but to get to zero.

Mike Wehner, now the assistant general manager at the Orange County Water District, runs the water purification program there, among much else. He has been involved with drinking water since 1971 when he went to work at the county health department. Wehner arrived at the Water District in 1991 to manage regulatory compliance, but his role has continually grown. Today, aside from his position at the Orange County Water District, he is a sought-after advisor by other utilities in the U.S. and around the world. For Wehner, his water utility is a part of the community's public health infrastructure, a worldview that should be standard, but isn't. Getting an organization devoted to pure, safe, and healthy water is, he says, a difficult and never-ending task.

"Our process begins even before the wastewater gets to the wastewater treatment plant," Wehner says. Since the purpose of the process is to get all dangerous chemicals out of the wastewater before it gets reused, the more toxic material that can be prevented from getting into the water, the easier it will be to clean. Orange County's sanitation department educates local businesses about proper disposal of materials that could get into the drain.[33] "It's more efficient and cheaper to screen contaminants at the source than later when contaminants have become widely dispersed, or combined with other chemicals, in the wastewater," Wehner says.

Another feature that makes Orange County special is that it has two separate sewer systems, one for collecting rainwater in the streets and a second one, that is called a sanitary sewer, for household sewage. While this isn't unique to Orange County, a majority of large and midsize American towns and cities—nearly eight hundred across the country—have sewer systems that combine the two. Most of the time, the combined sewers create no special problem. But when there is a larger than usual rainstorm, combined sewers often overflow. Instead of just rainwater backing up from the sewer, the combined overflow carries lots of contaminants like fecal matter to places where it poses a danger to the drinking water supply and to health. When you see a notice for closed beaches after a rainstorm, the reason is likely your community's combined sewer system. Orange County's bifurcated sewers prevents this problem.

Once sewage arrives in the Orange County wastewater treatment facilities, the initial phases of treatment are close to what is universally done in the U.S., even if it is performed in a technologically advanced and cost-efficient manner there. Items are filtered out with a series of screens. The remainder is allowed to sit with some small solids settling on the bottom of a tank and then removed. And then friendly bacteria are introduced to neutralize microorganisms and organic material, with the friendly bacteria also being removed after they have completed their work. Because the Orange County Sanitation District, which runs the county's wastewater treatment operations, is a partner in the reuse of water project, it has an interest in delivering "clean" treated sewage, both so that the final product is excellent quality and also to reduce costs.

It is here where Orange Country begins its differentiation from most everyone else. In nearly all other communities, the treated water at this stage meets federal and state guidelines and is legally permitted to be discharged into a public waterway like a river, lake, or ocean. But instead of disposing of the wastewater that way, the Sanitation District delivers the already-cleaned wastewater to the Groundwater Replenishment System.

At this point, Wehner says, the treated wastewater is drawn through microfilters. "This process removes tiny particles in the water that could pose a health risk," he says. "To give you a sense of scale of what we are talking about, the holes in these filters are invisible to the human eye.

They measure about 1/50,000th of an inch in diameter," or about 150 times narrower than the width of a single human hair. This filter removes any protozoa or bacteria, and also even some viruses that made it through the earlier wastewater treatment. "In addition," Wehner adds, "solids that have dissolved in the water can be filtered out at this first stage."

Following microfiltration, the already purer water is sent through a further round of cleaning by being pushed through reverse osmosis filters. The holes in these filters are about half the size of those in the microfilters. Reverse osmosis is the way that salt and minerals are removed from seawater in desalination. As with desalination, these filters remove salt and other minerals that may be dissolved in the water. But the filters do something more important than that.

"There are lots of residues of pharmaceutical compounds and other chemicals in wastewater," Wehner says. "These residues are removed by layers of filters bearing nano-sized holes. Any viruses that survived microfiltration also get trapped at this stage. The water that emerges from reverse osmosis filtration is so pure that it needs to have benign elements, like crushed limestone, added back in," which reduces acidity in order to prevent damage to the pipes used to transport the water.

In the final part of the ultra-purification process, the much treated water is exposed to ultraviolet light and hydrogen peroxide. "This not only serves to disinfect the water," says Wehner, "but also destroys organic compounds of a size and weight of a single molecule that may have made it through the reverse osmosis filtration. No biological element can survive this final treatment. All contaminants measured in the parts per trillion threshold are removed via this last step."[34]

At the end of this cleaning, the water is safe to drink. Visitors to the Groundwater Replenishment System are often given cups of water taken from a spigot at the end of a tour of this multi-phased cleaning. The water is just how you want water to look, smell, and taste. It is clear, odorless, and has no memorable taste. But the water isn't put directly into the county's water pipes, even if, no doubt, more than one city will soon super-cleanse its water in a sequence similar to this, and begin drinking it right away.

Each day, the Orange County Water District takes about 30 million gallons of this hyper-treated water and injects it into special wells used to rebalance the hydraulic pressure to keep the seawater out of Orange County's coastal aquifers. The remaining 70 million gallons (with 30 million gallons more to be added in 2022) are percolated into the county's groundwater. At a later time, this previously injected and percolated water is pumped out and used for homes and businesses. But even then, after it is extracted from the aquifer, the water is purified at the well-head once more, this time by chlorination.[35]

With the Groundwater Replenishment System, the people of Orange County get several benefits. They have protection from seawater intrusion which can ruin their aquifers and groundwater. They get a new source of water. The water the people of the county get through their taps is clean, healthy, and safe—and of higher quality than anything that comes from northern California or the Colorado River. And, most remarkably, in the middle of a dry region, due to the cycle of water purification and reuse that can be repeated indefinitely, they get to live as if they were in a wet region. Instead of the county's economic growth being put at risk, GWRS assures the residents there of all the water they could need or use.

As great as it is, the most valuable part of this process isn't the water that the people of Orange County get to drink. Rather, it is a model for us all that everything Orange County has done can be done with drinking water all over the U.S. Everyone can have tap water as clean and safe as the water Orange County produces.

How Orange County Became a Water Leader

Former California governor Jerry Brown made an astute observation years ago when he said, "There's no such thing as a free lunch." In popularizing a phrase used by economists, he was speaking then about the need for higher gasoline taxes to cover the cost of renovating and building new highways, but he could have been speaking about getting quality water into our homes and bodies. As with highways, there is no such thing as free water.

Most everyone prefers things at the lowest cost possible. But sometimes, cheap is the most expensive price, especially when the cheap item doesn't do the job it was bought to do. And when dealing with something that is irreplaceable—like health or the well-being of a loved one—avoiding cheap and less than perfectly cleaned water may be the best way to go. Add in peace of mind that abundance of water provides, and the water charges start to feel like a bargain.

The price of all of that Orange County water purification comes to an amount that may be too expensive for some, but not for most. Even assuming current technology doesn't get cheaper as it gets more efficient (which is usually the case), the cost of bringing all of the water to such a level of purity as enjoyed by Orange County is about $25 per person per year, including the cost of repaying all of the loans that were taken to build the system. If the value of all of the subsidies from the state and federal government were to be removed, the complete cost would rise to $33 per person per year, or about 63 cents a week.[36] With the price for reverse-osmosis-processed water dropping every few years as the technology gets better, these costs could stay stable or even decline.

These charges are in addition to existing water fees. But the existing expense of metering, wastewater treatment plants, and transporting water to consumers' homes are expenses that will exist regardless of water quality. Orange County also has expenses that most other places would not. Their water bills include the cost of the seawater barrier. Depending on the location and the needs of a community, costs could be even lower than in Orange County.

Other large communities could build similar facilities and assure peace of mind in quality and abundance of water at prices comparable to Orange County. Certainly, the source water for drinking water need not come from wastewater or seawater. Using the existing water supply would work as well in producing Orange County–quality drinking water, and presumably cleaner source water would make for yet cheaper treatment.

Smaller communities could not achieve the same efficiencies of scale, but could still be purifying their drinking water to a level better than the minimum quality required by the EPA. But even for these smaller communities, with the right incentives, lots of inventors could create purification systems for small population centers with outcomes similar to Orange County, and at favorable pricing. No one should have to have subpar-quality water because they live in small towns or rural communities.

Aside from the price necessary to be paid for reverse-osmosis-processed water, there are two arguments often made against using this technology. First, although it is becoming ever more energy efficient, reverse osmosis is energy intensive. It takes about the same amount of electricity to produce drinking water via reverse osmosis for a family of four as it does to run a standard home refrigerator. We don't give up our refrigerators, but at a time when efforts are being made to reduce energy usage, widescale use of reverse osmosis to clean drinking water creates a new demand for energy production. That said, there is no reason that the entire purification system here couldn't be run using power from a renewable grid. The Orange County Water District explored the use of solar power but found it would take decades before it would break-even on the current investment. It does, however, make use of other energy-saving devices in the purification process that reduce both cost and carbon fuels used.[37]

In addition, the contaminants removed from the water don't simply disappear. They have to be processed to be sure they don't return as a health hazard. Many communities put the toxic material in geologically safe landfills, but some send it to be incinerated and others—especially those adjacent to an ocean—have it carted to sea. GWRS takes the brine and all contaminants separated from the pure water, and transports it to the Orange County Sanitation District's ocean outfall where it is discharged into the Pacific Ocean. While this is certainly not ideal, it is no different from what currently happens with contaminants flushed down toilets and, after wastewater treatment, discharged to a waterway. Until a system of contaminant capture and reuse is instituted, this is likely to be the standard even in the most sophisticated wastewater and drinking water treatment plants.

In creating a water treatment system similar to the one in Orange County, admittedly, access to money makes a difference, and it isn't always available. But government loans and subsidies are provided more easily for projects where the stewards are knowledgeable and transparent in their use of public resources. Since repayment is often guaranteed by water fees, lenders know that their loans don't come with a lot of risk, especially if the borrower has a stable or growing population.

Funding for the GWRS and for other county water projects were available even during periods of statewide budget cutbacks or when the pendulum swung and public mood grew antagonistic to government taking on long-term spending obligations. During the creation of the GWRS, Orange County was then still one of the most politically conservative counties in mostly liberal California. Republicans held most local, state, and federal elective offices. Yet if Republicans are ideologically committed to smaller government budgets, Orange County's water projects were not a victim. Especially when the case is well presented, small-government conservatives prize quality drinking water no less than anyone else.

There is a reason that the Orange County Water District has won nearly every major water prize and why the county has a steady flow of visitors from around the U.S. and the world to see firsthand what they have done. It's worth asking why Orange County has been able to build out a water purification system of such quality while so many others continue to overtax existing water resources or to deliver water below an ideal quality.

While seawater intrusion into the freshwater aquifer was a powerful driver that started the investigations and experimentation that led to insights about water purification, the county has gone far beyond that. Likewise, it isn't fair to say that Orange County was driven by necessity or that they had no choice because water scarcity threatened their future, because other places face or faced growing fears of running out of drinking water, and either have done nothing or have waited far longer than they should have to take action.

The answer likely comes down to focus and desire. Since 1933 when the water district was founded—and long before the population boomed there—Orange County's officials made water quality and abundant supply a topic of central concern. It has never been an orphan issue without advocates and champions. Many places plan for no more than a few years ahead. In Orange County, there have been several water projects with a planned time line measured in decades, the most recent of which is the Groundwater Replenishment System. Mike Wehner is an heir to a tradition that aspires to the highest quality of water possible, and that sees complacency almost as great a threat as contaminated water is.

"It's impossible to say that we have achieved all that needs to be achieved," Wehner says. "Water quality is a continuous pursuit. We never know what is the next new contaminant. Since there are always new chemicals being invented, there are always things that we have to be thinking about. We have to constantly be on the lookout for the next challenge."

Mike Wehner has a theory as to why Orange County has achieved what so few others have in providing abundant, very safe water. It is an answer that might be called both practical and, in a sense, spiritual. "Our biggest advantage and the reason for our success," Wehner said, "is that we do all parts of the water process. We don't farm out anything. And we do everything because we have a sense of mission. You can ask anyone working here, and no one will say it's just another job. Working here is different from working at another public agency in some branch of the government. People here feel like they are building a cathedral. Something special and something that will last a very long time."[38]

Ten

NEW IDEAS NEEDED

*"If we put a public health emphasis on drinking water today,
it is hard to imagine all of the improvements in longevity and
quality of life we could have over the next fifty years."*
—Professor Jeffrey Griffiths, M.D.,
Tufts University School of Medicine

FIXING AMERICA'S DRINKING water system won't be easy, but it can
be done. If it is approached with vision and daring, it will change
life in America for the better over the next century and more. In addition to smarter laws, better regulation, and safer drinking water, a new
system for managing and providing drinking water will extend life expectancy and create many new business opportunities.

There is historical precedent that better drinking water can pay large
dividends. In the fifty years from 1900 to 1950, life expectancy in the
U.S. jumped by nearly 50 percent.[1] Without negating the role of advances
in medicine and lifestyle, economists at Harvard and Stanford special-
izing in health trends and demography concluded that the increase in life
span in the first half of the twentieth century was significantly tied to
the improvement in the quality of drinking water.[2]

Dr. Jeffrey Griffiths, a medical doctor and a professor of public health
at Tufts University, agrees with the economists' conclusion, but he takes

it a step further. "It takes fifty years for us to see the full benefit of the transformation of a water system," he says. "Because it happens so slowly, we are blind to how long this takes. If we put a public health emphasis on drinking water today, it is hard to imagine all of the improvements in longevity and quality of life we could have over the next fifty years."[3]

Aside from the greater individual personal satisfaction that healthier, longer lives would provide, Americans living and working longer—and spending less on health care—could produce a large benefit for productivity and the economy. With the possibility of more years at work, and also, among much else, more spending on homes, transportation, recreation, and tourism, national wealth would grow over the next several decades. Many new business opportunities would be created.

But the current mind-set in the drinking water industry and how it responds to new ideas is an impediment to achieving this transformation. It is not uncommon for industry veterans to oppose new engineering, technological, and organizational approaches that challenge the orthodoxy. Drinking water is a change-resistant industry, with an "If it ain't broke, don't fix it" worldview. That philosophy needs to be ended. If not, critical new technologies will be ignored in favor of the familiar when it comes time to replace existing operating systems. As technology infuses all other parts of our lives, it can happen in the world of drinking water, too. But innovators need to know that there will be a market for their ideas, or else they will put their efforts to work elsewhere.

The economic opportunity at hand may be the chance to start welcoming disruptive ideas. Globally, water is now a $700 billion business.[4] With water needs all around the world growing due to aged pipes, rising population, and a climate-change-induced need to augment water supplies, that number is certain to rise significantly. The fastest-growing parts of the water industry will be high-tech segments such as those that provide advanced water treatment, assure security, continuously monitor for water quality, and allow device-to-device wireless communication in pursuit of lower use of energy and reduction of water losses. Just as America has led the world in one important tech sector after another, the U.S. can be a global leader in water tech, driving progress and sales of U.S.-invented water innovations around the world.

To facilitate this, new federal and state policies can help spur new ideas and innovations. In Israel, surely the most advanced water tech country in the world, inventors with little more than a validated concept for a new water technology or an improvement on an existing one can receive government subsidies of 85 percent of their R&D budgets for the first two years of their new companies' lives. In addition, the best of those ideas are paired at no cost to the inventor with water utilities, providing a beta site for the concept. The utilities are given incentives to assist the inventors in fine-tuning their ideas. If the invention produces the desired result, it is soon adopted by other Israeli water utilities. From there, the inventor has a proven model with which to raise outside investment, and to begin selling around the world. This has resulted in a dynamic water tech industry that provides Israel with an abundance of high-quality drinking water in the driest region in the world. It has also generated billions of dollars in sales for Israeli water tech companies. One Israeli official estimates that—aside from the benefits to Israel's local and national water systems, and the high wage jobs it has helped to create—the incubator program has returned more than three dollars in new tax revenues for every dollar of R&D support provided by the Israeli government.[5] While developing better drinking water and better systems should be incentive enough, by adopting a system like Israel's that encourages innovation, the U.S. can create a new water tech sector with economic benefits that follow.

Another advantage of a well-run American drinking water system would likely be ending or lessening the need for bottled water, and with it, the extraordinary volume of disposable plastic drinking water bottles. At 70 billion individual containers a year (and growing), the rise of bottled water has produced mountains of trash at every landfill. With fewer than a quarter of the containers recycled and with the discarded bottles taking one hundred years or longer to decompose, our subpar drinking water has created an unintended second-order effect: a solid waste—and litter—problem.[6] But this can be reversed. Once public confidence returns to tap water, our environment and municipal budgets will be beneficiaries as the widespread use of disposable plastic drinking water bottles can be significantly reduced.

The effort to get better drinking water can also be a place where bipartisanship in Congress and state legislatures can be built, or rebuilt. There is no reason why safe drinking water shouldn't be a bipartisan issue. While many Republicans may have a skeptical view of environmental regulations, support for drinking water initiatives would benefit from being seen as a public health issue—as it was when the Safe Drinking Water Act was first passed in 1974 and strengthened with the 1986 Amendments with significant bipartisan support.

An argument can be made that better water policies already fit current Republican thinking. Republicans present themselves as the party of more efficient government. Consolidation of water utilities, more research into possible contaminants, empowering an innovative private sector in water tech, and prevention of disease are all compatible with Republican values. Further, with rural Americans who are served by a water utility suffering a large percentage of each year's Safe Drinking Water Act violations, it serves the interests of Republican elected officials to help get safer water and better health outcomes for a core group of their voters, as well as for all Americans.[7]

Another change that can improve drinking water would be for the uniformly communications-shy water utilities to begin doing consumer outreach. While consumers can't be expected to automatically embrace larger bills for their tap water or be pleased by disruptions from opening streets to replace pipes, ongoing consumer education will help. When the public understands the current state of drinking water—from an underinvestment in contaminant research, to the plethora of mostly underfunded water utilities, to why new pipes are needed—there will be more support for spending, water utility consolidation, and a more forgiving response to the temporary inconvenience of infrastructure-related construction.

Even well-run water utility officials often say that consumers would disapprove of water fees being spent on advertising, promotion, and non-essential communications. "If ratepayers see us marketing," says the head of one well-managed utility, "they will complain that if we have enough money for PR and awareness campaigns, we should cut water fees instead."

This creates a chicken-and-egg situation. Consumers can't be expected to understand the needs of a water system if they aren't informed about what it does and how it does it. In any event, not all outreach programs require an expensive campaign. Among other low-cost opportunities, every water utility should regularly schedule open-house tours to let locals learn about the water infrastructure that serves them; post online explanations of where consumers' water fees go; and recruit rotating volunteer citizens' advisory boards.[8] Local media should be encouraged to have a reporter whose responsibilities include covering water stories, and then—whether good news or bad—provide full access for each of those reporters. Then, when there is a need for a new water main or the replacement of all of the city's lead service lines, or for higher fees, consumers see themselves as part of the decision making. If still not eager to see costs rise, at least they understand where their money is going.

A few ideas follow on how to make drinking water better for us individually, for society as a whole, and for those in the generations to come. Some of these ideas call for large changes, others for simple ones, but all of them would alter the status quo. It isn't a comprehensive agenda, and is meant to only be a start.

More people pushing for change in drinking water are needed, and so are more ideas. Please share yours. How to do that follows at the end of this chapter.

Consolidate Water Utilities

America has too many water utilities. About 300 million Americans—everyone except for those who draw their water from a private well—get all or most of their drinking water from one of 51,535 water utilities.[9] For context, although there are 3,800 electric utilities in the U.S., fewer than 200 provide service for more than half of American homes and businesses.[10] Likewise, there are 450 U.S. cable TV and broadband service providers, but the top 10 of them provide service to more than 80 percent of all subscribers.[11] There are 435 congressional districts in the House of Representatives, with each congressperson representing about 710,000 people, while there is, on average, one water utility for every 55,300 users.[12] In the entirety of the U.S., there are 3,141 counties, which, on average, equals more than sixteen drinking water utilities per county.[13]

Having so many water utilities prevents millions of people from getting the best drinking water possible. It also wastes untold amounts of money from a range of inefficiencies caused by this redundancy. With so many small entities, it is impossible for them to create economies of scale that would be available with fewer, and larger, ones.

The bloated number of water utilities alone isn't the whole problem. Most of these small water utilities lack access to advanced technologies while being both under-resourced and understaffed. Few have the necessary reserve funds for emergencies or big projects. In all, 99 percent (the real number!) of America's water utilities provide drinking water to communities of 100,000 or less, with many of them serving only a few hundred people.[14] As a result, any benefit that a small size may bring in more hands-on customer service, ends up, unintentionally, working against the interests of the public they serve.

As discussed elsewhere in this book, the smaller the population that the utility serves, the lower its capacity, on average, to provide drinking water in compliance with its obligations under the Safe Drinking Water Act. But that's only the start of the problem: The law itself lowers the bar for these smaller entities. When it would be a financial hardship to do testing, small utilities are permitted to apply for an exemption from the EPA, which permits them to forgo testing for most contaminants. And when they do test and a contaminant is found, if they can show that eliminating or reducing that contaminant would be beyond either their current technical or financial capabilities, the EPA or the state allows them to defer an obligation to speedily address the problem. Although these variances and exemptions are intended to provide relief for smaller entities that are strapped for cash, in practice they may also be putting local populations at risk.

Further, small utilities have trouble attracting and retaining employees with high-level engineering skills, a particular problem as treatment of drinking water contaminants comes with ever greater technological challenges. And in addition, few of these utilities have financial reserves to help cover their share of the large replumbing of America's drinking water infrastructure that is coming. Meanwhile, most lack the expertise needed to borrow significant amounts of outside funding at reasonable rates to pay for major capital improvements. And with a shrinking subscriber base common in small communities, many of these water utilities might not be able to assure repayment, even if they could find a lender.[15]

While there is no magic number as to how many U.S. water utilities there should be, a goal of six to 12 per state, or a national total of 300 to 600, seems logical. Some geographically smaller states may need only one or two water utilities. Certainly, no state needs 7,500, as is the case with California—in which Los Angeles County alone has about 200 water utilities.[16]

With consolidation, economically poor areas would have access to capital and improvement in service while everyone's newly created water utility would benefit by increasing the base of customers. At the same time, significant savings would be realized by ending pointless duplication.

Caring for Rural America Means Caring for Private Wells

Forty-three million Americans get their drinking water from private wells.[17] Unlike in America's cities and suburbs, which are overwhelmingly serviced by water utilities, the EPA offers no assistance to those drinking private well water. Since most of these private water wells are located in rural areas, these communities are disproportionately shut out from getting water services.

The EPA doesn't require any kind of testing of private well water, and the Safe Drinking Water Act doesn't apply. There are no national regulations regarding how water from private wells should be treated to promote the optimal health outcomes. The EPA doesn't even offer criteria on how to manage a well and the water drawn from it. To avoid any doubt, the EPA website states: "Private well owners are responsible for the safety of their water."[18] As a result, millions of mostly rural dwellers are on their own when it comes to assuring safe drinking water.[19]

Likely the gravest problem created by this "Hear No Evil, See No Evil" approach by both federal and state environmental agencies is that rural water sources are being regularly contaminated. The best guess as to the pervasiveness of the problem was provided by a sampling of 2,167 wells—out of more than 13 million—in forty-eight states. But that research, done from 1991 through 2004 by the U.S. Geological Survey, is dated, providing a sense of how things were, but not likely as they are. Even so, the USGS concluded that nearly one in four of America's private wells suffer from chemical contamination at a concentration greater than what would be considered a safe level at a water utility.

At differing levels, 34 percent of the surveyed wells had E. coli and other bacterial agents in them and, although often at below current EPA-identified maximum contaminant levels, 60 percent had chemical elements including pesticides, refrigerants, and gasoline residues in the well water.[20] The variety of pollutants suggests that, aside from natural elements like arsenic or radon that widely get into these rural drinking water wells, the sources of contamination are agricultural, industrial, and domestic.

While not certain, it is likely that the degree of contamination is worse today than when the samples were taken from 1991 to 2004. But with the lack of federal oversight and regulations, and the very limited amount of data available, rural Americans are mostly left to guess how bad the situation may be and what the implications are for their health.

Feeding the suspicion that the problem is getting worse, a survey taken of three rural counties in Wisconsin in 2018 found that 42 percent of the wells inspected were contaminated with E. coli and a variety of agricultural contaminants.[21] Whether or not that small data set is predictive of a larger trend, it does reflect a significant increase in drinking well contamination over the earlier USGS research.

Because of the importance of agriculture in so many rural communities, it isn't surprising that one contaminant, in particular, is widely found in drinking water wells there. Nitrate contamination, derived from unabsorbed fertilizer and transmitted via groundwater, is the most common form of human pollutant found.[22] While there are programs from the Department of Agriculture to address nitrate contamination, they are targeted at preventing future nitrate runoff that would make the situation worse and not at remediating existing polluted wells.[23] In addition, a recent USGS study projects that as many as 2.1 million people using drinking water wells are being exposed to high rates of arsenic.[24]

Fracking has also been often suggested as a source of well water contamination. The practice of extracting oil and natural gas from rural areas has become an economic boon for many communities, with locals receiving royalties for the energy extracted from the earth below their property. But because of limited information on drilling mishaps, no one can be sure of the depth and breadth of contamination caused by these extractions.

There are approximately 975,000 fracking wells in the U.S. Since the 1970s when fracking began, there have been only a few hundred reported accidents and spills, and many of these reported incidents have not affected groundwater. In recent years, with better training and more safety practices in place, the number of *reported* accidents has dropped further. But the exact number of accidents, spills, or ruined drinking water wells from fracking is unknown.[25]

"When a fracking company contaminates someone's well," says Amy Mall, an expert on fracking who is a senior policy analyst at the NRDC, "they often quietly pay the owner of the well for the water they've contaminated, but we don't necessarily get details on the accident. Without comprehensive data collection, all we have is anecdotes and best guesses. The people in rural America deserve better. If we aren't regulating their drinking water wells under the Safe Drinking Water Act, which we should be doing, the least we could do would be to regulate fracking activity. If the drillers say it is safe to drill, they shouldn't have a problem having it regulated and requiring them to file reports on spills."

Speaking more generally about rural drinking water wells and not only about fracking, Mall adds, "If a family in rural America has lost the safe use of their well, they've lost everything. They can't sell their house, and, although some are economically secure and can move away, farm families are disproportionately poor or just getting by. They are smart and rugged people, but they are also among the most vulnerable to having their drinking water contaminated."[26]

Rural Americans should get the same opportunity for protection of their drinking water as city dwellers. Data should be collected as a basis for making policy. A federal agency should be available to assist in testing the well water of rural Americans and to offer ideas on removing contaminants.

Drinking Water Should Make a Major Technological Leap

The business of drinking water is a high-tech-deprived field. While the industry as a whole needs to do more to encourage new ideas and new technologies, three concepts, in particular, are worthy of attention and encouragement.

First, as America gets ready to replace much of the nation's drinking water infrastructure over the next two decades, pipe replacement will be a very large part of that. Rather than simply replacing an old steel pipe with a new one, the replacement pipes should be high-tech ones. Smart pipes can help to detect leaks, save on water lost, reduce energy needed to transport water, and report on conditions in the pipe. Choices made today will be imposed on the generations to come. Other parts of the drinking water infrastructure should also take a forward leap and be technologically advanced, but pipes installed now will be with us for as long as a hundred years, far longer than any control room hardware.

Second, as demonstrated in Orange County, especially at a time when the reuse of highly treated sewage for drinking and other purposes will become essential in populous, dry regions of the country, the very best systems should be put in place to make sure that drinking water is free of contaminants of all kinds. While wastewater treatment should jump a level and remove pharmaceutical residues, inorganic chemicals, and other contaminants to improve source water, it is even more important that advanced treatment techniques be universally adopted for drinking water.

Nanofiltration would be a great leap forward, but with the addition of ultraviolet and ozone treatments to the existing use of chlorine, everyone in fast-growing, water-scarce areas of the country could have a guarantee of contaminant-free tap water for less than a dollar a week per person more than what they are paying now—even when their drinking water is derived from a source as impure as sewage. This may start a virtuous circle: If water in Sun Belt communities can be treated to a perfect state of purity, Americans everywhere will be right to demand their water also be delivered to them free of contaminants.

A third technological innovation is also worth exploring, even if not completely ready for widespread adoption. Great progress has been made in the past few years with atmospheric water generation, drawing pure, uncontaminated drinking water out of the moisture in the air around us. Although there is always moisture in the air, it is especially present at night. And given that electricity prices drop after midnight, running the devices can be done with less-expensive energy that might otherwise go to waste. (Renewable energy sources could also power atmospheric water generators.)

These devices could be put on every house and apartment, and, by dawn, a day's worth of pure water for drinking and food preparation could be in the holding tank. Water from the water utility could be used for other household purposes like toilet flushing and lawn care, and in the community for firefighting. With use of atmospheric water generators, there would be no urgency in replacing lead service lines or installing reverse osmosis capabilities at drinking water distribution facilities. Pilot projects are already in place.[27] This is a technology that, if early tests perform as promised, may be ready for wide-scale adoption soon.

To learn more about how smart pipes, nanofiltration, reverse osmosis, ultraviolet and ozone treatment, and atmospheric water generators work, visit www.TroubledWater.US.

Move Drinking Water Out of the EPA

Companies routinely reorganize divisions to achieve better results. This happens less frequently at government agencies. But a rethinking of the EPA's jurisdiction over drinking water would likely yield important health benefits for all Americans.

With the passage of the Safe Drinking Water Act in 1974, the EPA was given responsibility for federal drinking water regulation. That decision may have made sense at the time when the EPA still saw itself as a part of the nation's public health infrastructure. But there was a change in outlook in the 1980s.[28] An ever-more bureaucratic EPA Office of Water is now less concerned with public health. The emphasis is now on cost-benefit analyses that measure threats from contaminants in drinking water versus the financial effect of regulating that water-borne pollutant.[29]

To recapture the original intent of regulating drinking water with public health primarily in mind, federal administration of drinking water should be removed from the EPA and relocated to the Department of Health and Human Services (HHS). The transition isn't assured of achieving better results. HHS may be subject to many of the same political constraints as the EPA. But if nothing else, the symbolic shock to the system of such a move would make clear to all that health is the top priority in federal administration of drinking water.

Ideally, the switch to HHS should be structured to insulate drinking water research from political pressure.[30] A freestanding scientific staff empowered to do what is in the best interest of America's health would produce the best outcomes. Funding should not be provided by Congress. Research and operations should be paid by a separate source of funding to protect against budget cutbacks motivated by an attempt to slow down this work. (See "Create a Well-Funded Independent Drinking Water Improvement Fund," immediately below.)

By being housed in HHS, the administration of drinking water would also benefit from being in close organizational proximity to other science-based agencies with responsibility for the nation's health. The Centers for Disease Control and Prevention (CDC), also under HHS, would be a worthy partner for drinking water's HHS-centered management. With the CDC's large research budget, funding for studies on the long-term health effects of a range of chemicals in drinking water would make sense, and be money well spent. In addition, the health research arm of the federal government, the National Institutes of Health, and in particular the National Institute of Environmental Health Sciences, reside in HHS and would be an important sister organization for the drinking water program.

For the reorganization of drinking water from the EPA to HHS to succeed, Congress will have to restrain the often quiet machinations of the president's Office of Management and Budget. Under presidents of both parties, the OMB has repeatedly interfered with actions planned by the EPA to regulate drinking water contaminants. This has happened especially—but not only—when the Pentagon or another federal department or agency is responsible for the contamination.[31]

Similar to the federal structure, each of the 50 states has an agency devoted to the environment in which significant jurisdiction of drinking water falls. As with the benefit of moving responsibility for drinking water out of the EPA and over to HHS, states would also be better off having drinking water administered by a health-centric government organization.

Dr. Mona Hanna-Attisha, the pediatrician and scientist in Flint, Michigan, whose data made clear that children were being harmed by the elevated lead levels in drinking water, believes that the Flint crisis would have been avoided had state drinking water decision making been made by scientists and doctors concerned about public health. "When it comes to safeguarding the health of the public, no level of government—whether federal, state, or local—gets it right," she says. "The denial and delay that we got from the [Michigan] Department of Environmental Quality would never have occurred had jurisdiction of drinking water been centered on where public health would be best protected."

Create a Well-Funded Independent Drinking Water Improvement Fund

The hunt for contaminants in drinking water and their potential health effect is too slow and greatly underfunded. While the federal budget is opaque and drinking water research is found in several places, the vast majority of EPA water research funding goes for surface water under the Clean Water Act and not for drinking water under the Safe Drinking Water Act. For the 2019 (fiscal year) federal budget, slightly less than $3.6 million is budgeted for dedicated drinking water research.[32] One industry expert says his best "guesstimate" is that the aggregate U.S.

spending of all independent, non-industry-funded drinking water contaminants research is no more than $15 million a year.[33] With new chemicals regularly coming to market, there is no way at current funding levels to keep up with the inventory of compounds that should be reviewed or tested.

It is obvious that the sooner a chemical is studied, the quicker its safety or danger can be known. It has also been the general experience of the EPA and researchers in hydrochemistry that the more intensively a known dangerous contaminant is studied at different levels of concentration, the quicker an appropriate safe level can be set for it. Proving the point, several contaminants that have had their safe level set by the EPA have later had it set lower following further study.[34]

One impediment to drinking water research that should be removed is a lack of funding. Drinking water safety is too important to be without necessary resources. And the money shouldn't be a hostage to the whims of Congress and state legislators. Research dollars should come from fees, and all funds generated should go into a locked box trust fund administered by a scientific advisory board, independent of Congress.

There are many potential sources of independent drinking water research funding. Here are two, one originating from bottled water, and the other from tap water.

Last year, more than 70 billion disposable drinking water containers were used in the U.S.[35] Several states assess a bottle fee of five to ten cents that is kept if the bottle isn't returned for recycling. Some communities also charge a per ounce tax on carbonated beverages as a revenue source, supposedly to fight obesity or litter, but these taxes mostly go into the general budget.[36]

A two-cent per disposable bottled water container federal tax would yield $1.4 billion each year. It would be collected from whoever produces drinking water containers.

Likewise, there is a very large amount of tap water used every day in the U.S. The U.S. Geological Survey estimates that (not including water used for agriculture) the average American uses between 80 and 100 gallons of water a day for all purposes, with lawn watering, toilet flushing, and bathing being the leading three.[37] Multiplied by the U.S. population, that comes to 355 billion gallons per day. Multiplied by 365 days, the vast amount of total water used tallies up to a number with many zeroes.

If a federal tax of, say, one penny per thousand gallons were to be assessed, it, too, would yield resources of over a billion dollars each year.

No one would notice the two cents per bottle or the penny per thousand gallons of tap water, but—paid into a federal drinking water improvement fund—it would provide all of the resources needed to allow chemists to study contaminants. These modest taxes could also be used to accelerate research into promising new water-purification technologies, or for independent inspectors sampling drinking water for contaminants, or for a variety of other valuable safe drinking water-centric activities.

Amend the 1996 Amendments

There should be a significant overhaul of the Safe Drinking Water Act, with a special emphasis on repealing the worst of the 1996 Amendments. In particular, the EPA (or, if transferred, HHS) should be obliged to more aggressively identify drinking water contaminants. As important, the time horizon for deciding on whether to regulate a contaminant should be shortened. Additionally, the extraordinarily complex set of analyses required for regulation of contaminants must be substantially streamlined. The law should return to the pre-1996 approach requiring standards to be set based on protecting public health to the degree that is feasible rather than allowing endless arguments about costs and benefits to tie the process in knots. While perchlorate is an extreme example at more than twenty years of review without a conclusion, no contaminant should be under consideration for more than a few years without the agency coming to a decision. When in doubt, a more protective standard should be adopted.

During the (long) wait to see if a contaminant should be regulated, consumers aren't permitted to bring a lawsuit against a water utility under the Safe Drinking Water Act regarding that contaminant or any unregulated toxic element. Congress should remedy this by allowing consumers to sue their utilities if any health risk is found in the drinking water—even if it is not a regulated contaminant. This change will incentivize better procedures and more protection, and would likely encourage water utilities and local governments to take a more active role in understanding what is in their water. Moreover, to the extent that the EPA now acts at all in regulating a contaminant, it is for wide-scale threats with national implications. Removing this immunity from lawsuit for water utilities would help to localize a solution, as it would help to protect people from the often overlooked risks present in local communities.

The 1996 Amendments also put a limit on how much research the EPA is permitted to do into drinking water contaminants.[38] A better approach would be to not only expect the EPA—or whichever body ultimately oversees drinking water—to study as many contaminants as the agency believed should be studied (without an arbitrary and artificial cap of thirty), but to press that government agency or department to step up the pace of its research.

One other immediate change would be worthwhile. The Consumer Confidence Reports created by the 1996 Amendments were supposed to enhance transparency and promote consumer education.[39] But they are mostly incomprehensible. Few people look at them. A revised law should require water utilities to clearly explain the contaminants found and the risks they present, and to present information about contamination and violations available online in real time. Consumers will demand more when they understand more.

Take Testing Off the Honor System

The system created by the EPA to check for the presence of lead and other contaminants in drinking water wasn't formally designed to encourage cheating or erroneous results, but it might as well have been. Under an honor system, each water utility selects how, where, and when to sample. In the worst case, it encourages dishonest practices by water utilities. And even if the water utilities intend to act with full integrity, the current system allows for the taking of samples by staff that may lack the technical skills or training to be sure that the surveys are being done properly. Either way, the reliability of the results is threatened.

The failure to properly sample, which can result in the under-reporting of contaminants, can create a false sense of security. By providing underestimates of risk, the public may have less concern than it should about the quality of its drinking water. And then, because the public believes there is no reason to be concerned, individuals have no reason to learn more, or to demand professional testing. Better sampling yielding honest results can provide either the impetus for improvement of drinking water supply or consumer confidence that they can drink from their tap without worry.

Lead testing, which is done in a limited number of homes in each municipality, is likely to provide erroneous results most of the time. Instead of "first-liter" testing now done by homeowners, professional samplers should be drawing multiple samples. When handled professionally, high lead levels will often be detected in later-drawn samples, even when first-liter-drawn samples had displayed no presence of lead.

The solution is to have samples taken by highly skilled, independent samplers at both the drinking water central distribution facility and in randomly selected homes. In the case of contaminants such as lead that are known to hit certain homes or areas hardest, testing should be required at those locations at highest risk. Samplers should only be driven by the timely development of the most accurate data.

As an alternative, and where the technology exists for individual contaminants, the EPA should compel an end to manual monitoring and transition to continuous automated sampling and testing. This is another example of how the water utilities have failed to use available technology to provide better quality water.

Regardless of how the monitoring is done, all test results should be promptly made public by the lab—and with no interference by the water utility—in an easy-to-understand format that is searchable online.

Water Vouchers for the Poor

Everyone deserves high-quality water. Unfortunately, even at current prices, drinking water is still too expensive for many low-income households. As a result, every year millions of Americans have their taps shut off by their water utility for nonpayment. In 2016, an estimated 15 million people in nearly five million U.S. households suffered this inconvenience, disruption, and humiliation.[40] Reconnection fees can be significant, especially when interest and penalties on the unpaid water bills are added in.

Not surprisingly, those most likely to have their water shut off are poor. Yet we don't allow poor people to go without food and, although there are those suffering from homelessness in every city, we see it as a national, state, and local responsibility to get most poor people into housing. Welfare assistance also helps to augment available funds for life's necessities like clothing and shoes. Medicaid provides a medical safety net for the very poor.

Despite the many ways in which indigent Americans are provided with material support, only about 30 percent of cities offer water assistance to low-income households.[41] No one should have to go without water for drinking, food preparation, washing, and sanitation. Water vouchers should be available for the poorest in every community. Instead of it being an everyday affair, shutoffs by water utilities should be rare. Those less well-off should pay what they can for their water, even if that is less than the real cost, but it should be everyone's right to have access to safe and affordable water.

More Ideas Are Needed

The use of drinking water is the only interaction that every American is guaranteed to have with their government every day. Even so, there are not enough people talking about drinking water, and there are too few ideas in circulation on what to do to improve the quality of it. Every popular movement has begun with the coalescing of new approaches to problems.

To help encourage a national conversation about drinking water and what should be done, a sharing of ideas is essential. To sign up to learn more about drinking water technologies, or to share your ideas or your reaction to ideas in this book, get in touch at www.TroubledWater.US.

Let's get the drinking water we deserve.

Eleven

WHAT YOU CAN DO NOW

*"Let's say I'm not willing to wait five or ten years for a solution.
What can I do right now to get safer water?"*
—Dr. Liron Friedman,
environmental engineer

IT IS POSSIBLE to imagine a day when everyone in America who is thirsty can fill a glass of water from a sink and have no reason to wonder about the quality of the water or to worry about what drinking it might do to their long-term health. We know what has to be done.

But that day is not here. We now drink from that sink because that is the water that is available. Yet, the more you know, the more unsettled you may feel. That sense that we can have better water may move many to push for a reform of drinking water in America.

In the meantime, while waiting for Congress and the EPA to act and while advocating for a systemic change in our approach to drinking water, it is wise to do what we can to protect ourselves and our families immediately by drinking the best quality water we can get. As Dr. Liron Friedman said after reading the manuscript for this book, "Let's say I'm not willing to wait five or ten years for a solution. What can I do right now to get safer water?" Likely, many readers had the same thought.

The good news is that there are a variety of ways for everyone to improve the quality of their drinking water. These solutions may not be as good, as inexpensive, or as beneficial for society as it would be if done on a national scale, but better is better. And until every person getting their water from a drinking water utility or from a private drinking water well has safe water to drink and with which to prepare food, it may be best—while still moving as quickly as possible on systemic change—to address this fixable problem on a house-by-house and sink-by-sink basis.

So, what should a person do to get that better drinking water right now?

Here are a few actions that can help those who want to have more peace of mind and better drinking water almost immediately.

Know Your Surroundings

Some places are more prone to drinking water contaminants than others. As such, having information about your neighborhood and the place where you live is important.

For example, if you live in a high-rise apartment building, you aren't likely to be getting much lead in your drinking water. Lead service lines can't handle the water pressure needed for a volume of water that large. On the other hand, if you live in a private home built before 1991 or in an apartment building of five or six stories or smaller, you may be getting your water via lead pipes.

Likewise, if your home is connected to a septic system and you get your drinking water from a private well, it is important to get your water tested. A variety of contaminants may be migrating from a leaky septic tank to your well via groundwater. While it is helpful to have your septic system inspected for leaks every five years, if you get municipal water, there may be contaminants in it, but it isn't coming from your septic system.

Beyond your own home, pay attention to what is going on in your neighborhood. If there is construction or road work or if you live on a street on which heavy trucks regularly travel, anti-corrosion compounds in the pipes providing water to your home may be shaking off. If so, it is wise to test for lead and, while waiting for the results, to switch to bottled water.

And casting an eye farther than your front steps and the street in front of you, try to find out if there are chemical factories within three miles of your home. If so, note that you may be living in what is sometimes called a "fenceline" community. Homes within fenceline communities are at greater risk of air and water pollution. It is worthwhile to ask your local government environmental agency what inspections they do to assure that such factories are using the highest safety standards and are not currently in violation of regulations that could put your drinking water at risk.

If you are unsure about what might be in your water, the best way to know is by testing it. There are home tests available for sale on the internet to test for lead and bacteria ($69). But if you fear you may have PFOA, perchlorate, heavy metals (like arsenic, chromium, copper or manganese, among others) or other more complex contaminants, a home test isn't as easy to do. Sometimes, local water utilities will provide this testing for free. Check with your local water utility. If not, you will have to send out samples to a lab. These are also easy to find on the internet, but—as important as it is to get testing done—be forewarned that many of these tests can run as much as a few hundred dollars for each contaminant tested.

Read the Consumer Confidence Report

One of the supposed victories for better drinking water came with the 1996 Amendments to the Safe Drinking Water Act. It required each drinking water utility to prepare an annual Consumer Confidence Report in which information about local drinking water quality is provided. Unfortunately, these reports have failed to achieve what was intended. They are confusing—possibly deliberately so—and most people discard them without reading, seeing the form as a worthless government notice easy to ignore. Among its other flaws, the reports focus on regulated contaminants, and do not give a complete profile of what else might be in the water.

These criticisms are valid. Congress and the EPA should mandate a better form. But until that happens, even if incomplete and cumbersome, the Consumer Confidence Report can be a useful tool for a partial understanding of your drinking water. Ask your local water utility for a copy of the report for your area. Try to read it, but if you can't understand what you are looking at, don't give up. Call the water utility and ask the customer service representative to explain it to you in nontechnical language. You have a right to know.

If You Are a Farmer (or Live Near One)

People living in rural America may often have less pure drinking water than their cousins in cities. If you are a farmer (or live near one) and get your drinking water from a private well, there is a reasonable chance you will find a number of dangerous contaminants in your drinking water. As referenced in the last chapter, the EPA has no oversight on private water wells and offers no assistance. You are on your own.

Some states offer advisory services, and, when available, you should make use of them. In any event, whether handled by a state agency or not, drinking water wells should be tested every year or so for a variety of contaminants. Although these tests can be expensive, once you know what contaminants are in your drinking water, you can buy appropriate treatment technologies to protect yourself and your family. Without that information, you are forced to guess as to whether you have tainted water. The insight that a test provides can enhance your family's health and provide you with peace of mind. A basic test for E. coli and nitrates is $139, but advanced testing that includes a search for industrial chemicals and heavy metals can cost $650 and more.

But regardless of what the tests reveal, you can also take steps to protect your water from new contaminants or denser contamination from existing ones.

If you are raising animals, make sure that manure pits on your farm are lined and sealed. Animal waste often gets into groundwater and from there into water wells. Stopping E. coli from getting into drinking water on farms can be done with this as a protective measure.

Likewise, if you grow crops, be mindful on use of pesticides, herbicides, and fertilizer. They can all get into the groundwater and, again, find their way into your drinking water. Contact your local state agricultural extension office to learn what you can do to reduce runoff with pollutants. Many have funding from the U.S. Department of Agriculture or can offer incentive payments from downriver water utilities to install systems on your farm that protects both people living in those communities and you.

If you test your well water and find contaminants or even if you suspect they are there, use drinking water filters of the kind discussed below.

Bottled Water

Bottled water was described elsewhere in this book as an alternative drinking water system. It will be a good day when everyone can be certain that their tap water is of such quality that bottled water will not be considered as an alternative for it. But realistically, that day is not here.

All bottled water is alike in that it comes in a disposable container. Despite that similarity, there is a wide variation in quality within the many hundreds of bottled water products available for sale. (See Chapter 5.) While no bottled water is certain to be pure—the plastic alone can be a source of contamination—some of them are likely to be of higher quality than others. Without making an endorsement, bottled water brands from protected sources (such as Fiji and S.Pelligrino) are likely to have fewer contaminants, at trace levels or otherwise. Some domestic brands that are tap water but which have gone through nanofiltration or reverse osmosis (such as Aquafina and Dasani) are also likely to be of a higher quality.

Of singular concern, though, and as discussed in the chapter on plastic, is how the plastic bottle was shipped and stored at every stage, from bottling to final sale to you. If left in a warehouse or outdoors with high temperatures, especially if it was done for several days or longer, contaminants from the bottle can leach into the drinking water. Similarly, after purchasing the bottled water, it is important to not leave the bottles in a heated car or to store them in direct sunshine where, again, leaching may occur.

Safe Reusable Bottles

To keep hydrated, if you have an active lifestyle and prefer to travel with your own water container, make sure you do what you can to protect yourself. First, know what material was used to manufacture your bottle. Some reusable plastic is likely benign, but others have demonstrated leaching of harmful or questionable chemicals. Although they are legally offered for sale, it is prudent to stay away from BPA plastic bottles. Unlined stainless steel bottles are probably the safest choice. Don't assume a bottle is safe just because you can buy it at a reputable store. While it would be nice to think that a government agency or your retailer has investigated the safety of the material before it has gone on sale, it may not be so.

Although it may seem obvious, pay heed to what water you are using to fill your reusable container. Since the range of quality is so different, if possible, fill up from a source you have reason to know is safe.

Wash your reusable bottle daily. Bacteria from your mouth and from your surroundings can get into the bottle and grow. Even stainless steel bottles (which are naturally anti-bacterial) can develop colonies of bacteria. And if you do choose to use a reusable plastic bottle, as with disposable plastic bottles, don't leave your durable plastic bottle in a hot place, such as a closed car in the summer. Many bacteria thrive in such tropical microclimates.

In Your Home

With so many Americans concerned about the quality of the water in their home, many products have been developed to handle some or all of the concerns. The price range is significant, as is the quality of outcome.

The easiest to use and the least expensive of these products are pitchers with activated carbon filters ($25 to $60). Gravity pulls the water through the filter. The carbon in the filter chemically bonds with many contaminants, and removes them from the drinking water. Since none of these pitchers remove all of the possible contaminants, it is important to read the product description and decide what kind of protection you are seeking. At its most basic, pitcher filters get rid of chlorine and the unpleasant taste that comes with it. But there is a large variety of pitcher filters for a wide variety of contaminants. These come from well-known brands including Brita, PUR, DuPont, and ZeroWater, as well as many others.

While the brand may provide assurance of manufacturing quality, the filter is only effective if it is matched to the contaminant needing to be removed. Also, it is very important to change the filter approximately every forty gallons or else the filter will either be ineffective or could be a source of contamination.

Slightly more expensive, faucet filters ($27 to $79) are attached to the faucet in a sink. The principle of how it works is similar to pitchers, except the water pressure from the faucet drives the water through the activated carbon. Most faucet filters require no tools or expertise for installation. Culligan and PUR, among other brands, sell faucet filters.

The filters last longer than for pitchers, providing up to 200 gallons of purified drinking water.

Yet more expensive, and possibly requiring professional installation, are under-sink filters ($75 to $250). These filters are connected to the water supply under the kitchen sink and are connected to either the regular faucet or a dedicated line. Under-sink filtration systems are offered by several well-known companies including Kohler and Aquasana. These devices can filter a large amount of water to a relatively high level of purity, and with a low per gallon cost.

If you enjoyed high school chemistry, you may prefer to set up a distillation system in your kitchen. These units use tap water. The water is boiled and the vapor condenses on a closed surface. As the vapor cools, it changes from a gas (steam) back to a solid (water), and the water is directed into a collector. What is collected is pure water, with all chemicals and other contaminants left behind to be poured down the sink. A distillation system can be put together from household items such as a large pot, a lid and a bowl, but countertop distillation machines are for sale, with a wide price range ($87 to $599) depending on volume of water and other features.

The most expensive of all home purification products is reverse osmosis, also called RO. It comes in two forms: One purifies drinking water from a specific faucet and the other purifies all of the water used in the house for all purposes. Both take up a significant amount of space, require professional installation, and require expensive equipment (as much as $4,000). Reverse osmosis systems force water through nano-sized filters, removing all contaminants, leaving only pure water behind. As a negative, they also use a lot of electricity, and require a lot of water to operate. Reverse osmosis units require between five and twenty gallons of water for every gallon of usable water produced. Sink systems are usually installed in the kitchen so that the pure water can be used for drinking and food preparation. Whole house systems are installed at the point where the water comes from the service line into the house. For both systems, filters need to be changed no less often than annually, and replacement is best done by a professional, adding expense to these choices.

A person of means may say that if reverse osmosis is best and if the house has the necessary space for installation, no other choice makes sense. But it is possible to see it from a more practical perspective. It your water or well is comprehensively tested every year, you can know what contaminants are present and buy a filter appropriate to the problem. In some cases, that may result in a reverse osmosis system, but if a simple pitcher filter provides the same outcome, it may not be worth the cost, the extra use of electricity, and wasted water. Even so, a reverse osmosis system is as close to a guarantee as you can get that all contaminants have been removed.

Into the Future

Imagine a day when none of the concerns or water filters will be necessary. On that day, if you are thirsty, you will just go to the sink and turn on the tap. You will fill your glass with what is guaranteed to be contaminant-free water, and drink. It is possible. It is what we should demand.

Acknowledgments

Writing a book is supposed to be a lonely, solitary affair, but I met so many interesting, inspiring, and helpful people in the course of the research and writing of this book that I never felt as if this were a solo venture. Instead, I saw myself as a weaver of a tapestry in a busy workshop where everyone added a guiding touch.

Above all, thanks goes to the ninety-one people—eighty-five of them listed at the end of these Acknowledgments—who took time to speak with me and to share their views of the state of drinking water and how to make it better. I learned something (and usually, many things) from each of them, and only my concern about producing an overlong book kept me from quoting every one of them. In one way or another, the wisdom imparted from each of them shaped my views here and is reflected in these pages.

Several people currently working in government or at a water utility were very helpful, but asked to not be identified. Although I can't list them by name, my appreciation is even greater for their help. Several of them appear as anonymous sources in the book, something I'd prefer to not have had to do, but their insights were too valuable not to include.

Even though everyone I interviewed gave so much to the final product, a few deserve special mention. Ronnie Levin, a wise, passionate, and very funny person, spent many hours over three long interviews speaking with me about lead, the EPA, the water utility industry, and much more. She also turned over a filing cabinet full of reports and news clips about lead and water she has acquired over many years. In what was probably the shortest interview, Jeff Griffiths shared his vision for a better drinking water system that has inspired me ever since. Likewise, Hank Habicht, who has spent most of his life working to provide better, safer water for all, offered many wise insights worthy of a book of his own. John Doyle's life story and his description of his work on behalf of the Crow people was the most moving experience I had while working on this book. Judith Enck told me about Hoosick Falls and shared all of her contacts and files. David LaFrance, G. Tracy Mehan III, and Greg Kail generously spent a lot of time in interviews and follow-up emails, providing fascinating insights from the industry point of view that added balance and perspective to my understanding. Diana Aga, Luke Iwanowicz, Melanie Marty, Mike Schock, Veena Singla, and Martin Wagner are all serious scientists who were able to get even a liberal arts type like me to understand the science that has been their respective life works and the risks before us. They (and Professor Paul Milazzo, and Bill Romanelli, too) also read sections of the manuscript to correct errors of both nuance and fact.

No one is due more thanks than Erik Olson, who sat through enough interviews to fill a few of my notebooks with his thoughts. The depth of his knowledge is remarkable, as is the breadth of his concern for the public's well-being. Although it is certain that he has strongly held beliefs, this modest and soft-spoken leader never once tried to convert me to his views. A perfect teacher, he systematically explained the world of drinking water, leaving me to draw my own inferences.

I was also fortunate to have more than a few people I admire volunteer to read drafts of the book. Thank you to Sam Adelsberg, Richard Banks, Antony Currie, Liron Friedman, Scott Harris, Dan Polisar, Peter Rup, Alana Siegel, and Sam Siegel. Every one of them shared ideas that made the book better, sometimes causing me to discard sections, chapters, and, a few times, the entire structure of the book. In addition to her important help with the look of the book cover, Talia Siegel played an indispensable role in the design and development of www. TroubledWater.US, the website that accompanies this book. Thank you, also, to Caroline Siegel, who, in the midst of seemingly endless nights working as a medical resident, took time to send suggestions for possible book titles. Josh Schildkraut also helped with marketing advice. Each of them are busy people. The time and focus they put into reading and advising awes and inspires me.

After writing *Let There Be Water,* I wasn't sure if I wanted to commit to another book, and, if so, what the topic should be. Marcia Markland, my editor at Thomas Dunne Books on that book, convinced me to try another water book. Although she is no longer at the publishing company, she remains a friend. I am fortunate that, in her place, Tom Dunne assigned the wise and diligent Stephen S. Power to be my editor. The final product is so much better for his gentle touch. And a special word of thanks to my agent, Mel Berger of WME, who read drafts and has been a believer in the potential of this book as both an important story to tell and as an agent of change.

Very special thanks are due the Daniel M. Soref Charitable Trust—a visionary organization devoted to the common good—for bringing me together with the University of Wisconsin–Milwaukee's School of Freshwater Sciences. In addition to my serving as the Daniel M. Soref Senior Policy Fellow at the School while writing this book, the Trust also generously arranged funding for the School to provide a research assistant—Katie Hall—for this project. It is difficult to convey Katie's passion for this topic, her integrity, her work ethic, or her upbeat personality. If I am lucky, she will stay with me for water books to come. Not a day goes by when she doesn't teach me something new about the world of water and unearth some source that perfectly makes the point. I am also fortunate to have become warm friends with the kind and generous people involved with the Trust.

Perhaps strangely, I'd also like to thank someone who had nothing to do with this book. Dr. Dan Lieber was a complete stranger when *Let There Be Water* was published. Passionate about its message, he arranged for policymakers and academics around the world—and many of his patients and friends, too—to have a copy of the book. Along the way, he became my friend and my partner in building awareness of Israel's solutions for water scarcity.

Finally, I'd like to thank my family, and especially my wife, Rachel Ringler. I suspect I've shared a few too many water stories with them over the past few years, but they have always listened with good cheer. I dedicate this book to Rachel—my partner, best friend, wife, and the kindest person I have ever known—whose wisdom and beauty still captivate me after a lifetime together—and to our children, with thanks for the never-ending joy and love they inspire.

INTERVIEW LIST

(Titles shown are accurate as of the time of the interview)

NOTE: For different reasons, some of those interviewed wished to be anonymous. Since that "Not for Attribution" requirement allowed them to speak candidly, their names do not appear here.

John Adams—Cofounder and former CEO, Natural Resources Defense Council

Diana Aga—Professor, Chemistry, State University of New York at Buffalo

Dror Avisar—Professor, Hydrochemistry, and Director, Water Research Center, Tel Aviv University

Edo Bar-Zeev—Senior Lecturer, Zuckerberg Institute for Water Research, Ben-Gurion University

Mitch Bernard—Chief Legal Officer, Natural Resources Defense Council

Earl Blumenauer—U.S. Congressman

Adam Bosch—Head of Public Affairs, New York City Department of Environmental Protection

Peter Bower—Senior Lecturer, Environmental Science, Barnard College

Barbara Boxer—Former U.S. Senator

Irene Caminer—Director of Legal Services, Chicago Department of Water Management

Kartik Chandran—Professor of Earth and Environmental Engineering, Columbia University

Albert Cho—Vice President, Strategy and Business Development, Xylem Inc.

Jennifer Clary—Water Programs Manager (California), Clean Water Action

Ken Cook—President and Cofounder, Environmental Working Group

Bill de Blasio—Mayor, City of New York

Greg Dotson—Assistant Professor, University of Oregon School of Law; former Chief Staffer for Energy and Environmental Policy, Congressman Henry Waxman

John Doyle—Co-Director, Apsaalooke Water and Wastewater Authority; Member, Crow Nation Environmental Steering Committee

Marc Edwards—Professor, Environmental and Water Resources Engineering, Virginia Tech University

Jim Elder—Former Director, EPA Office of Ground Water and Drinking Water

Marti Emerald—Former consumer affairs reporter, KGTV–San Diego, and former San Diego City Council member

Judith Enck—EPA Region 2 Administrator

Dave Engel—Attorney, Village of Hoosick Falls; former Attorney, Healthy Hoosick Water; Of Counsel, Nolan & Heller

Jay Famiglietti—Professor, Earth Science Systems, University of California, Irvine; Senior Water Scientist, NASA Jet Propulsion Laboratory

Maureo Fernández y Mora—Drinking Water Advocate (Massachusetts), Clean Water Action

Alex Formuzis—Director of Communications, Environmental Working Group

Kathryn Garcia—Interim Chair, New York City Housing Authority and Senior Advisor, Citywide Lead Prevention

Eric Goldstein—Senior Attorney and New York City Environment Director, Natural Resources Defense Council

Bill Goodman—Town Supervisor, Ithaca, New York

Igal Gozlan, PhD—Senior Analytical Chemist, Water Research Center, Tel Aviv University

Jeffrey Griffiths—Professor, Public Health and Medicine, Tufts University School of Medicine

Charles "Chip" Groat—Former Director, U.S. Geological Survey

Hank Habicht—Former EPA Deputy Administrator and Chief Operating Officer

Dr. Mona Hanna-Attisha—Director, Pediatric Public Health Initiative, Michigan State University and Hurley Children's Hospital

Michael Hickey—Resident, Hoosick Falls

Luke Iwanowicz—Research Biologist, U.S. Geological Survey

Greg Kail—Director of Communications, American Water Works Association

Mike Keegan—Legislative Director, National Rural Water Association

Rebecca Klaper—Professor, School of Freshwater Sciences, University of Wisconsin–Milwaukee

Greg Koch—Senior Director, Global Water Stewardships, Coca-Cola

David LaFrance—CEO, American Water Works Association

Ronnie Levin—Visiting Scientist, Harvard School of Public Health; Former Senior Scientist, EPA Office of Environmental Stewardship

Brendan Lyons—Editor and Reporter, *Albany Times Union*

Alex MacDonald—Senior Water Resource Control Engineer, California Water Resources Control Board

Amy Mall—Senior Policy Analyst, Natural Resources Defense Council

Felicia Marcus—Chair, State Water Resources Control Board (California)

Michael R. Markus—General Manager, Orange County Water District

Marcus Martinez, MD—Resident and local physician, Hoosick Falls

Melanie Marty, PhD—Deputy Director, Scientific Affairs, California Office of Environmental Health Hazard Assessment

Jan Matuszko—Chief, Engineering and Analytical Support Branch, EPA Office of Water

G. Tracy Mehan III—Executive Director, Government Affairs, American Water Works Association

Martin Melosi—Professor, History, University of Houston

Pat Mulroy—Former Director, Southern Nevada Water Authority

Barrett Murphy—Commissioner, Chicago Department of Water Management

Olga Naidenko, PhD—Senior Science Advisor, Environmental Working Group

Tom Neltner—Chemicals Policy Director, Environmental Defense Fund

Jonathan Nichols—Associate Research Professor, Lamont-Doherty Earth Observatory, Columbia University

Pam Nixon—Former Environmental Advocate, State of West Virginia

Erik Olson—Senior Director, Health and Food, Healthy People and Thriving Communities Program, Natural Resources Defense Council

Dr. David Ozonoff—Professor, Environmental Health, Boston University School of Public Health

Bettina Poirier—Professor, American University Washington College of Law; former Chief of Staff, Senator Barbara Boxer

James Proctor—Senior Vice President and General Counsel, McWane, Inc.

Abby Reneger—Professor, Halmos College of Natural Sciences and Oceanography, Nova Southeastern University

Bruce Reznik—Executive Director, Los Angeles Waterkeeper

Michele Roberts—National Co-coordinator, Environmental Justice Health Alliance

Bill Romanelli—Spokesperson, Perchlorate Information Bureau

Michael Schock—Scientist, Office of Research and Development, U.S. Environmental Protection Agency

Joel Schwartz—Professor, Environmental Epidemiology, Harvard School of Public Health

Gerald A. Silver—Founder, Homeowners of Encino; Professor Emeritus, Los Angeles City College

Veena Singla—Professor and Associate Director, Program on Reproductive Health and the Environment, University of California, San Francisco

Velma Smith—Former Executive Director, Friends of the Earth

J. Gustave Speth—Cofounder, Natural Resources Defense Council

Shanna Swan—Professor, Environmental Medicine and Public Health, Mount Sinai College of Medicine

Nelson Switzer—Chief Sustainability Officer, Nestlé Waters North America

Joel Tarr—Professor, History, Carnegie Mellon University

Forest Tennant, MD and PhD—Former Mayor, West Covina, California

Patricia (Patsy) Tennyson—Executive Vice President, Katz & Associates; Advisor, San Diego County Water Authority

Lynn Thorp—Director, National Campaigns, Clean Water Action

Eleanor Torres—Director, Public Affairs, Orange County Water District

Martin Wagner—Associate Professor, Biology, Norwegian University of Science and Technology

Henry Waxman—Former U.S. Congressman

Mike Wehner—Assistant General Manager, Orange County Water District

Andrew J. Whelton—Associate Professor, Civil, Environmental, and Ecological Engineering, Purdue University

Peter Williams—Consultant, Waterfind USA

Claire Woods—Staff Attorney, Natural Resources Defense Council

Thomas Zoeller—Professor, Biology, University of Massachusetts–Amherst

Notes

ONE: WELCOME TO HOOSICK FALLS!

1. "Timeline: Town of Hoosick 1900–2000," Hoosick Township Historical Society, compiled by Gilbert E. Wright, Town Historian, 1995–1999, accessed October 31, 2018: http://www.hoosickhistory.com/shortstories/timeline2000.htm.

2. At one point, there were 675 jobs in eleven different factories making Teflon in Hoosick Falls. Michael Hickey, author's interview, February 16, 2017.

3. Michael Hickey, author's interview, February 26, 2017.

4. For a history of 3M Company, see *A Century of Innovation: The 3M Story* (Maplewood, MN: 3M Company, 2002).

5. Speech of Joseph H. Simons, given on July 19, 1973, found in "The Seven Ages of Fluorine Chemistry," *Journal of Fluorine Chemistry* 32 (1986): 7–24.

6. PFOA is only one of several chemicals developed from Professor Simons's original invention that fall into what are called PFAS, a diverse group of chemical compounds that are resistant to heat, moisture, and grease. PFOS, another compound in that group, was long used as a firefighting foam. PFOS has been shown to be responsible for an array of diseases and birth defects.

7. Anna McCarthy, *The Citizen Machine: Governing by Television in 1950s America* (New York: The New Press, 2010), 45–50.

8. Robert Friedel, "The Accidental Inventor," *Discover* 17, no. 10 (October 1996): 58–69.

9. Susan Feyder, "3M Takes Friendly Rival DuPont to Court over Licensing Fees," *Star Tribune*, April 22, 2010.

10. US Environmental Protection Agency, *Drinking Water Health Advisory for Perfluorooctanoic Acid, EPA 822-R-16-005* (Washington, DC: US Environmental Protection Agency, Office of Water, May 2016): 14.

11. "About Gore: Applications of ePTFE: Fluoropolymer Fibers," Gore, accessed 10/31/18: https://www.gore.com/about/technologies/applications-fluoropolymer-fibers.

12. Granta Y. Yakayama, Assistant Administrator, "Consent Agreement and Proposed Final Order to Resolve DuPont's Failure to Submit Substantial Risk Information Under the Toxic Substances Control Act and Failure to Submit Data Requested Under the Resource Conservation and Recovery Act," Memorandum to the Environmental Appeals Board, US Environmental Protection Agency (December 14, 2005), 2.

13. PFOA can be incinerated but only under very well-controlled conditions and at extremely high temperatures, 2,000° F. At lower temperatures, incineration of PFOA will usually result in release into the air. Elisabeth L. Hawley et al., *Remediation Technologies for Perfluorinated Compounds (PFCs), Including Perfluorooctane Sulfonate (PFOS) and Perfluorooctanoic Acid (PFOA),* White Paper, London, UK: ARCADIS, May 2012.

14. C. W. Fetter, *Applied Hydrogeology,* 4th edition (Harlow, England: Pearson Education, 2014), 427–33.

15. Ian Ross et al., "A Review of Emerging Technologies for Remediation of PFASs," *Remediation* 28, no. 2 (March 12, 2018): 101–26.

16. "PFOA in Drinking Water 2016," Vermont Department of Health, accessed December 22, 2018: http://www.healthvermont.gov/response/environmental/pfoa-drinking-water-2016.

17. See Steven Johnson's *The Ghost Map,* a chilling but exceptionally well-told story about Dr. John Snow and his methodical effort at figuring out the locus of a cholera epidemic in Victorian London. *The Ghost Map: The Story of London's Most Terrifying Epidemic and How It Changed Science, Cities, and the Modern World* (New York: Riverhead Books, 2007).

18. In 1849, President James Polk died of cholera shortly after leaving office. In 1862, Willie Lincoln, the son of Abraham Lincoln, died in the White House of typhoid fever from water supplied to the presidential residence. Peter Ilyich Tchaikovsky, the celebrated Russian composer of *The Nutcracker* and *Swan Lake,* died in Saint Petersburg in 1893 of cholera, nine days after the premiere of his Sixth Symphony.

19. The deadly pathogen Cryptosporidium is often immune from treatment with chlorine and requires advanced treatment such as ultraviolet light (UV) for maximum protection. Since a large number of U.S. drinking water systems do not use UV or other of these techniques, death by Cryptosporidium remains a real possibility in much of the country. For the effectiveness of UV, see J. L. Zimmer et al., "Inactivation and Potential

Repair of *Cryptosporidium Parvum* Following Low- and Medium-Pressure Ultraviolet Irradiation," *Water Research* 37, no. 14 (August 2003): 3517.

20. The presence of unwanted chemicals and pathogens that survive the treatment process in drinking water don't always take decades, or even many years, to manifest their danger. Lead in any concentration interferes with the neurodevelopment of fetuses, babies, young children, and possibly even teenagers. Likewise, there are dangerous pathogens like Cryptosporidium and Legionella, among others, that can sicken or kill within days of drinking water containing them. The Centers for Disease Control and Prevention estimates that there are 13 million cases of "waterborne illness due to contaminated municipal source water systems (public drinking water distributed by the water utility)." See "Healthy Water: Current Waterborne Disease Burden Data & Gaps," Centers for Disease Control and Prevention, Division of Foodborne, Waterborne and Environmental Diseases, accessed August 9, 2017: https://www.cdc.gov/healthywater/burden/current-data.html.

21. Nathaniel Rich, "The Lawyer Who Became DuPont's Worst Nightmare," *New York Times,* January 6, 2016.

22. PFOA is one of many chemicals in the fluorine family that were created from the initial intuition of Professor Joseph Simons in the 1930s and 1940s. The author's choice to focus on PFOA is not intended to suggest that it is uniquely dangerous or that it is the only member of the perfluoroalkyls, or PFAS, that is worthy of study and regulation. In particular, PFOS seems to pose a significant threat to human health. The Agency for Toxic Substances and Disease Registry's 2018 report on perfluoroalkyls makes clear what has been known for some time: These chemicals—transmitted via water, air, food, and/or soil—may be a threat to public health. Agency for Toxic Substances and Disease Registry, *Toxicological Profile for Perfluoroalkyls, Draft for Public Comment* (Atlanta: US Department of Health and Human Services, June 2018).

23. Ironically, given that it was the report of Isabel McGuire's melanoma that set off Michael's initial internet hunt, McGuire's melanoma was more likely to have been caused by her work for many summers as town lifeguard than due to PFOA-related contamination.

24. Marcus Martinez, author's interview, February 26, 2019.

25. Dave Engel, author's interview, February 26, 2019.

26. Brendan Lyons, "Saint-Gobain Coaches Mayor," *Albany Times Union*, May 8, 2016, and Brendan Lyons, "Saint-Gobain, Hoosick Falls Officials Worked Closely, Emails Reveal," *Albany Times Union*, May 9, 2016.

27. *Safe Drinking Water Act Amendments of 1996,* 42 U.S.C. 300f–300j, as amended by P.L. 104–182, "Unregulated Contaminants," §1445 (42 U.S.C. 300j-4).

28. Ibid., "Small System Variances," §1415 (42 U.S.C. 300g-4).

29. "Monitoring Unregulated Drinking Water Contaminants: Fourth Unregulated Contaminant Monitoring Rule," US Environmental Protection Agency, accessed December 8, 2018: https://www.epa.gov/dwucmr/fourth-unregulated-contaminant-monitoring-rule.

30. The Environmental Working Group has identified 172 sites with contaminated drinking water due to PFAS and estimates that more than 1,500 drinking water systems, serving up to 110 million Americans, have been affected. "Update: Mapping the Expanding PFAS Crisis: Known Contamination from Toxic Fluorinated Chemicals Keeps Spreading, with No End in Sight," Environmental Working Group, accessed October 15, 2018: https://www.ewg.org/research/update-mapping-expanding-pfas-crisis.

31. Marie J. French, "Hoosick Falls Residents Angered by Proposed Settlement with Saint Gobain, Honeywell," *Politico,* January 12, 2017.

32. Dave Engel, author's interview, February 26, 2019.

33. Brendan Lyons, "A Danger That Lurks Below," *Albany Times Union,* December 14, 2015.

34. Brendan Lyons, author's interview, October 8, 2018.

35. Judith Enck, author's interview, June 21, 2016.

36. Brendan Lyons, "Invoices Detail Hidden Legal Work in Hoosick Falls," *Albany Times Union*, April 26, 2017; Brendan Lyons, "Hoosick Falls Secretly Hired GE Consultant for Pollution PR," *Albany Times Union*, January 22, 2016.

37. Brendan Lyons, email to the author, December 22, 2018. As a result of Lyons's report, the arrangement was cancelled. Some legal fees were paid, but Lyons believes the public relations firm decided to not bill Hoosick Falls for the services rendered.

38. Jesse McKinley, "Fears About Water Supply Grip Village That Made Teflon Products," *New York Times,* February 28, 2017.

39. Philippe Grandjean and Richard Clapp, "Changing Interpretation of Human Health Risks from Perfluorinated Compounds," *Public Health Reports* 129, no. 6 (November–December 2014): 482–85; Philippe Grandjean and Richard Clapp, "Perfluorinated Alkyl Substances: Emerging Insights into Health Risks," *New Solutions* 25, no. 2 (June 17, 2015): 147–63.

40. Agency for Toxic Substances and Disease Registry, *Toxicological Profile for Perfluoroalkyls, Draft for Public Comment,* 15–16.

41. The earliest use of activated carbon as a filter goes back to antiquity. Egyptians and Sumerians began using it around 3,750 BCE. Ferhan Çeçen, "Water and Wastewater Treatment: Historical Perspective of Activated Carbon Adsorption and Its Integration with Biological Processes," in *Water and Wastewater Treatment: Integration of Adsorption and Biological Treatment Integration,* edited by Ferhan Çeçen and Özgür Aktas (Weinheim, Germany: Wiley-VCH Verlag, 2011), 1.

42. Michael Hickey, email to the author, November 30, 2018.

43. Michael Hickey, author's interview, March 10, 2018.

TWO: THE EPA TAKES CONTROL OF DRINKING WATER

1. Michael J. McGuire, *The Chlorine Revolution: Water Disinfection and the Fight to Save Lives* (Denver: American Water Works Association, 2013), 111–13.

2. Although Maidstone, England, was the first instance of chlorine being used for a community, in a variant chemical form it was also used as a disinfectant for drinking water during a typhoid epidemic at an Austro-Hungarian naval base in Pola in 1896. See J. B. Rose and Y. Masago, "A Toast to Our Health: Our Journey Toward Safe Water," *Water Science and Technology: Water Supply* 7, no. 1 (2007): 41–48.

3. Stephen Johnson, *The Ghost Map: The Story of London's Most Terrifying Epidemic and How it Changed Science, Cities, and the Modern World* (New York: Riverhead Books, 2007), 213–15.

4. Jay Gould and Jim Fisk, "Belden Millions to Go to Family: Court Throws Out Assignment Giving Interest in Jersey Water Supply Co. to His Brother," *New York Times,* July 15, 1910.

5. McGuire, *The Chlorine Revolution: Water Disinfection and the Fight to Save Lives,* 220–21.

6. Ibid., 133.

7. Ibid., 226.

8. Ibid., 252.

9. Ibid., 257.

10. The Centers for Disease Control and Prevention (CDC) tracks waterborne illness in the U.S. Even in good years, there are several hundred thousand reports of emergency room visits from tainted water that lead to further hospitalization and even death. Despite chlorination and filtration, in 1993 about 400,000 people in Milwaukee—half of the city's population—was sickened by Cryptosporidium, resulting in as many as 100 deaths. See William R. Mac Kenzie et al., "A Massive Outbreak in Milwaukee of Cryptosporidium Infection Transmitted Through the Public Water Supply," *The New England Journal of Medicine* 331, no. 3. (July 21, 1994): 161–67; and also, regarding death toll, see "Cryptosporidium in Milwaukee's Water Supply Caused Widespread Illness," *Infectious Disease News* (September 2007). In 2008, the CDC estimated that there were approximately 19.5 million waterborne illnesses annually in the U.S., even if only a small percentage ended in hospitalization and a yet smaller number resulted in death. See "Current Waterborne Disease Burden Data and Gaps: 2008 Estimates," US Department of Health and Human Services, Centers for Disease Control and Prevention, accessed August 9, 2017: https://www.cdc.gov/healthywater/burden/current-data .html. All that said, the horror of cholera epidemics has been all but eliminated as a concern in the developed world.

11. McGuire, *The Chlorine Revolution: Water Disinfection and the Fight to Save Lives,* 127–28.

12. James Symons, "The Early History of Disinfection By-Products: A Personal Chronicle—Part 1," *Environmental Engineer* 37, no. 1 (January 2001): 21–25.

13. *Safe Drinking Water Act,* 42 U.S.C. 300f–300j (1974).

14. So deep was the water utilities' antagonism to the passage of the Safe Drinking Water Act that it was a widely held belief among those in the industry that the chlorine-THM link was a scam driven by a conspiracy to get the law passed. See Symons, "The Early History of Disinfection By-Products: A Personal Chronicle—Part 1," 25.

15. States and territories have the right to opt out of participating in the Safe Drinking Water Act. Only Wyoming and Washington, D.C., have done so, leaving administration to the EPA. In all other cases, states receive a small annual payment in exchange for serving as administrator in their state.

16. A few states, especially California and Massachusetts, came to develop sophisticated programs to identify and control contaminants, but most rely on the EPA for direction in these areas.

17. After President Nixon's veto, the Senate and House voted 52–12 and 247–23, respectively, to override the veto. See E. W. Kenworthy, "Clean-Water Bill Is Law Despite President's Veto," *New York Times,* October 19, 1972.

18. Henry Waxman, author's interview, January 30, 2018.

19. Jim Elder, author's interview, April 16, 2018.

20. Erik Olson, email to the author, September 10, 2018.

21. Ronnie Levin, author's interview, April 25, 2018.

22. Email to the author, confidential source, August 28, 2017.

23. Henry Waxman, author's interview, January 30, 2018.

24. Jim Elder, author's interview, April 16, 2018.

25. Henry Waxman, author's interview, January 30, 2018.

26. Diane VanDe Hei and Thomas Schaeffer, "SDWA: Looking to the Future," *Drinking Water Regulation and Health* (New York: John Wiley & Sons, 2003), 115.

27. US Environmental Protection Agency, *National Primary Drinking Water Regulations, EPA 816-F-09-004* (Washington, DC: US Environmental Protection Agency, May 2009).

28. VanDe Hei and Schaeffer, *Drinking Water Regulation and Health,* 116. See also Kenneth F. Gray, "The Safe Drinking Water Act Amendments of 1986: Now a Tougher Act to Follow," *Environmental Law Reporter* 15 (1986): 10338–45.

29. *Safe Drinking Water Act Amendments of 1986,* 42 U.S.C. 300f–300j, as amended by P.L. 99–339, §1412 (b) (2) (A-B).

30. Ibid., §1412 (b) (3–8).

31. Ibid., §1417.

32. Henry Waxman, author's interview, January 30, 2018.

33. Ronald Reagan, *Statement on Signing the Safe Drinking Water Act Amendments of 1986,* June 19, 1986.

34. In a 2018 poll, 88 percent of those polled supported more *federal government* spending on water problems. See "Third Annual Value of Water Index," US Water Alliance, Value of Water Campaign, accessed November 30, 2018: http://thevalueofwater.org/resources.

35. Jim Elder, email to the author, September 18, 2018.

36. VanDe Hei and Schaeffer, *Drinking Water Regulation and Health,* 117.

37. This claim was made despite the authority that Congress gave to the EPA to substitute up to seven contaminants that posed a greater health risk than those on the list of toxic substances identified in the legislation. *Safe Drinking Water Act Amendments of 1986,* §1417.

38. US General Accounting Office, *Drinking Water: Compliance Problems Undermine EPA Program as New Challenges Emerge, GAO 90–127* (Washington, DC: US General Accounting Office, June 8, 1990); and US General Accounting Office, *Drinking Water: Widening Gap Between Needs and Available Resources Threatens Vital EPA Program, GAO 92–184* (Washington, DC: US General Accounting Office, July 6, 1992).

39. Erik Olson, author's interview, February 13, 2018.

40. Henry Waxman, author's interview, January 30, 2018.

41. *Safe Drinking Water Act Amendments of 1996,* 42 U.S.C. 300f–300j, as amended by P.L. 104–182, "State Revolving Loan Funds," §1452 (42 U.S.C. 300j-12 [m]).

42. Ibid., "Unregulated Contaminants," §1445 (42 U.S.C. 300j-4).

43. Greg Dotson, author's interview, February 26, 2018.

THREE: AN ENDLESS ROAD TO NOWHERE

1. As discussed later in the chapter, since individual states are permitted to have standards higher than those of the EPA, the decisions of California and Massachusetts to regulate perchlorate creates a requirement that water utilities in those states must reduce the concentration of that chemical in the drinking water they provide.

2. Tom Neltner, "Little Follow-Up When FDA Finds High Levels of Perchlorate in Food," *Environmental Defense Fund,* November 2, 2017.

3. 42 U.S.C. 300g-1(b)(1)(C) an (b)(3)(C)(i)(V).

4. Philip J. Landrigan and Lynn R. Goldman, "Children's Vulnerability to Toxic Chemicals: A Challenge and Opportunity to Strengthen Health and Environmental Policy," *Health Affairs* 30, no. 5 (May 2011).

5. Clayton W. Trumpholt et al., "Perchlorate: Sources, Uses, and Occurrences in the Environment," *Remediation* (2005): 68.

6. Agency for Toxic Substances and Disease Registry (ATSDR), *Public Health Statement on Perchlorates* (Atlanta: US Department of Health and Human Services, September 2008), 1.

7. Trumpholt et al., "Perchlorate: Sources, Uses, and Occurrences in the Environment."

8. Presentation by Dr. David Kimbrough, "Sunset Reservoir Wells Perchlorate Investigation—Sources of Perchlorate," April 30, 2013. Presented to the US EPA at the Jet Propulsion Laboratory, Pasadena, CA.

9. US Environmental Protection Agency, *Perchlorate Environmental Contamination: Toxicological Review and Risk Characterization, External Review Draft, NCEA-1-0503* (Washington, DC: US Environmental Protection Agency, Office of Research and Development, January 16, 2002), E2.

10. The space shuttle boosters all use solid-fuel rockets, and these make use of perchlorate as an oxidizer. But the Apollo Saturn V rocket—the most powerful one ever launched— was a liquid-fueled rocket that used liquid oxygen as an oxidizer and contained no perchlorate. See Agency for Toxic Substances and Disease Registry (ATSDR), *Public Health Statement on Perchlorates,* 2.

11. Interstate Technology and Regulatory Council (ITRC), *Perchlorate: Overview of Issues, Status, and Remedial Options* (Washington, DC: ITRC, September 2005), 9.

12. Trumpholt et al., "Perchlorate: Sources, Uses, and Occurrences in the Environment," 83.

13. John Stanbury and James Wyngaarden, "Effect of Perchlorate on the Human Thyroid Gland," *Metabolism* 1, no. 6 (November 1952): 533–39.

14. Angela M. Leung et al., "Perchlorate, Iodine and the Thyroid," *Best Practice & Research: Clinical Endocrinology & Metabolism* 24, no. 1 (2010): 133–41.

15. US Government Accountability Office, *Perchlorate: A System to Track Sampling and Cleanup Results Is Needed, GAO-05-462* (Washington, DC: US Government Accountability Office, May 20, 2005), 20–21.

16. Alex MacDonald, author's interview, March 15, 2018.

17. Kathleen Sellers et al., *Perchlorate: Environmental Problems and Solutions* (Boca Raton, FL: CRC Press, Taylor and Francis Group, 2007), 18–23.

18. Richard Dahl, "Perchlorate Debate Grows," *Environmental Health Perspectives* 112, no. 10 (July 2004): A546.

19. Igal Gozlan, author's interview, February 6, 2017.

20. "Fentanyl: What Is a Lethal Dose?," Oxford Treatment Center, accessed December 4, 2018: https://www.oxfordtreatment.com/fentanyl/lethal-dose/.

21. "Fentanyl Patch Can Be Deadly to Children," US Food and Drug Administration, February 23, 2013.

22. Ronald A. Hites, "Dioxins: An Overview and History," *Environmental Science & Technology* 45, no. 1 (2011): 16–20.

23. E. Thomas Zoeller et al., "Endocrine-Disrupting Chemicals and Public Health Protection: A Statement of Principles from the Endocrine Society," *Endocrinology* 153, no. 9 (2012): 4097–4110.

24. Elizabeth N. Pearce et al., "Consequences of Iodine Deficiency and Excess in Pregnant Women: An Overview of Current Knowns and Unknowns," *The American Journal of Clinical Nutrition* 104, no. 3 (September 2016): 919S.

25. Thomas Zoeller, author's interview, November 2, 2018.

26. R. Thomas Zoeller, "Collision of Basic and Applied Approaches to Risk Assessment of Thyroid Toxicants," *Annals New York Academy of Sciences* (2006): 168–77.

27. R. Sobhani et al., "Process Analysis and Economics of Drinking Water Production from Coastal Aquifers Containing Chromophoric Dissolved Organic Matter and Bromide Using Nanofiltration and Ozonation," *Journal of Environmental Management* 93 (2012): 209–17.

28. In December 2006, the European Union enacted *Registration, Evaluation, Authorization and Restriction of Chemicals* (REACH), establishing a European chemical agency and a process for evaluating new chemicals being introduced. Unlike the *Toxic Substances Control Act* in the U.S., REACH is governed by the principle "No data, No market," meaning the chemical manufacturer must provide data that illustrates that the chemical is safe before it is allowed to be produced. EC 1907/2006. However, for the imperfect implementation of this EU rule, see Anton Lazarus, "Precautionary in Principle, Flawed in Fact: European Commission Review Accepts Environmental Groups' Criticism of Chemical Regulation," European Environmental Bureau (EEB), March 6, 2018.

29. *Toxic Substances Control Act*, §4.

30. Veena Singla, author's interview, June 18, 2018.

31. Rena Steinzor, *Mother Earth and Uncle Sam: How Pollution and Hollow Government Hurt Our Kids* (Austin: University of Texas Press, 2008), 128.

32. Alex MacDonald, author's interview, March 15, 2018.

33. Pat Mulroy, email to the author, July 10, 2018.

34. For more information on the history of the Hoover Dam and Lake Mead, see the US Bureau of Reclamation, "The Story of the Hoover Dam—Essays," accessed December 18, 2018: https://www.usbr.gov/lc/hooverdam/history/essays/essays.html; and Michael Hiltzik, *Colossus: Hoover Dam and the Making of the American Century* (New York: Free Press, 2010).

35. In 1930, the southwestern states had the following populations: Arizona—435,573, New Mexico—423,317, Nevada—91,058, and California—5,677,251 (US Census Bureau, *US Census 1910,* vol. 1 [1910]: 27). The Hoover Dam was completed in 1935. In 1980, the southwestern states had the following populations: Arizona—2,718,215, New Mexico—1,302,894, Nevada—800,493, and California—23,667,902. US Census Bureau, *Summary of the United States, Table 8: Population 1790—1980* (Suitland, MD: US Census Bureau, 1980), I-43.

36. Michael R. Rosen et al., *A Synthesis of Aquatic Science for Management of Lakes Mead and Mohave: U.S. Geological Survey Circular 1381* (Reston, VA: US Geological Survey, 2012), 1.

37. Pat Mulroy, author's interview, March 14, 2018.

38. U.S. Food and Drug Administration, *2004–2005 Exploratory Survey Data on Perchlorate in Food* (Silver Spring, MD: US Food and Drug Administration, 2006); and U.S. Food and Drug Administration, *Survey Data on Perchlorate in Food—2005–2006 and 2008–2012 Total Diet Study Results* (Silver Spring, MD: US Food and Drug Administration, 2014).

39. Pat Mulroy, author's interview, March 14, 2018.

40. "How EPA Regulates Drinking Water Contaminants," US Environmental Protection Agency, accessed November 20, 2018: https://www.epa.gov/dwregdev/how-epa -regulates-drinking-water-contaminants.

41. *Comprehensive Environmental Response, Compensation, and Liability Act (CERCLA),* 42 U.S.C. §9601 et seq. (1980).

42. The few exceptions to this are the Unregulated Contaminant Monitoring Rule (*Safe Drinking Water Act Amendments of 1996,* "Unregulated Contaminants," §1445 (42 U.S.C. 300j-4)). In addition, a few states, such as California, Massachusetts, and New Jersey, require additional monitoring and, in rare cases, treatment beyond federal requirements.

43. Jennifer 8. Lee, "Second Thoughts on a Chemical: In Water, How Much Is Too Much?," *New York Times,* March 2, 2004.

44. US Government Accountability Office, *Perchlorate: A System to Track Sampling and Cleanup Results Is Needed.*

45. Hank Habicht, author's interview, October 26, 2018.

46. Erik Olson, author's interview, March 2, 2018.

47. The EPA made the final regulatory determination to not regulate twenty-four contaminants from the Contaminant Candidate Lists. Additionally, the EPA has decided that two other contaminants meet the standard for regulation under the Safe Drinking Water Act—perchlorate and strontium. Regulatory Determination 1 decided that nine contaminants would not be regulated (Federal Register, vol. 68, no. 138, July 18, 2003). Regulatory Determination 2 decided that eleven contaminants would not be regulated (Federal Register, vol. 73, no. 147, July 30, 2008). Regulatory Determination 2 decided

that four contaminants would not be regulated and one, strontium, would be considered for regulation (Federal Register, vol. 81, no. 1, January 4, 2016). Note that, as with perchlorate, the EPA has delayed a regulation decision on strontium; in this case, to evaluate the effects of treatment technology.

48. US Government Accountability Office, *Perchlorate: A System to Track Sampling and Cleanup Results Is Needed,* 20–21.

49. Craig Steinmaus et al., "Thyroid Hormones and Moderate Exposure to Perchlorate During Pregnancy in Women in Southern California," *Environmental Health Perspectives* 124, no. 6 (2016): 861–67.

50. US Environmental Protection Agency, *Perchlorate Environmental Contamination: Toxicological Review and Risk Characterization (External Review Draft).*

51. National Research Council, *Health Implications of Perchlorate Ingestion* (Washington, DC: National Academies Press, 2005), 22.

52. The Natural Resources Defense Council (NRDC) filed several Freedom of Information Act requests, ultimately having to file lawsuits to get many of the requested documents. The federal government opposed the NRDC effort to reveal what was proposed at that meeting. See Erik Olson and Jennifer Sass, "White House and Pentagon Bias National Academy Perchlorate Report," Natural Resources Defense Council, January 10, 2005; and *Natural Resources Defense Council v. United States Department of Defense,* 442 F.Supp.2d 857 (2006).

53. Jennifer Sass, "U.S. Department of Defense and White House Working Together to Avoid Liability for Perchlorate Pollution," *International Journal of Occupational and Environmental Health* (2004): 330–34.

54. Drinking Water: Preliminary Regulatory Determination on Perchlorate, 73 Federal Register 60274, October 10, 2008.

55. Letter from Melanie Marty, Chair, EPA Children's Health Protection Advisory Committee, to Stephen L. Johnson, US EPA, March 8, 2006.

56. Drinking Water: Preliminary Regulatory Determination on Perchlorate, 73 Federal Register 60262–60282, October 10, 2008.

57. US Government Accountability Office, *Perchlorate: A System to Track Sampling and Cleanup Results Is Needed.* Although perchlorate was found in drinking water sampled in twenty-eight states, it was also found in soil samples in an additional seventeen states. This raises the possibility that private drinking water wells are also contaminated with perchlorate. Drinking water wells are not monitored by the EPA. The EPA statement can be found at US Environmental Protection Agency, *Fact Sheet: Preliminary Regulatory Determination for Perchlorate, EPA 815-F-08-009* (Washington, DC: US Environmental Protection Agency, Office of Water, October 2008).

58. Juliet Eilperin, "EPA Makes No Rule on Chemical in Water," *Washington Post*, October 4, 2008.

59. *Safe Drinking Water Act Amendments of 1996,* "National Drinking Water Regulations," §1412, (42 U.S.C. 300g-1(b)(2)).

60. Transcript, *Natural Resources Defense Council, Inc. v. United States Environmental Protection Agency, et al.,* Conference before Hon. Edgardo Ramos, District Judge, United States District Court, Southern District of New York (August 31, 2016), 5.

61. Consent Decree, *Natural Resources Defense Council v. Environmental Protection Agency, Case No. 16-cv-1251,* United States District Court for the Southern District of New York, October 18, 2016.

62. Philip Brandhuber et al., "A Review of Perchlorate Occurrence in Public Drinking Water Systems," *Journal of the American Water Works Association* 101, no. 11 (November 2009): 64.

63. US Environmental Protection Agency, *Technical Fact Sheet—Perchlorate, EPA—505—F—7—003* (Washington, DC: US Environmental Protection Agency, September 2017), 4.

64. Melanie Marty, author's interview, April 4, 2018.

65. Ibid.

FOUR: PILLS IN THE WATER

1. National Center for Health Statistics, *Health, United States, 2016: With Chartbook on Long-term Trends in Health,* Table 79 (Hyattsville, MD: US Department of Health and Human Services, 2017), 293–94.

2. Ibid., Table 80.

3. US Centers for Disease Control and Prevention, *Antibiotic Use in the United States, 2017: Progress and Opportunities* (Atlanta: US Department of Health and Human Services, 2017), 15.

4. "National Drug Code Directory," US Department of Health and Human Services, Food and Drug Administration (FDA), accessed October 10, 2017: https://www.fda.gov /Drugs/InformationOnDrugs/ucm142438.htm.

5. There are 305,510 pharmacists in the U.S. See "Occupational Employment and Wages, May 2016, Pharmacists," US Bureau of Labor Statistics, accessed August 29, 2017: https://www.bls.gov/oes/current/oes291051.htm. There are 61,009 pharmacies in the U.S. See National Community Pharmacists Association, *NCPA 2016 Digest: Opportunities for Community Pharmacy in a Changing Market* (Alexandria, VA: NCPA, 2016), 9. 3.7 billion drug prescriptions were ordered as a result of physician office visits, and 340.6 million drug prescriptions were ordered as a result of hospital emergency department visits. See National Center for Health Statistics, *National Ambulatory Medical Care Survey:*

2015 State and National Summary Tables (Hyattsville, MD: US Department of Health and Human Services, 2015), Tables 21–26. 329.2 million drug prescriptions were ordered as a result of hospital outpatient department visits. See National Center for Health Statistics, *National Ambulatory Medical Care Survey: 2011 Outpatient Department Summary Tables,* Tables 18–20.

6. Suzanne M. Kirchhoff et al., *Frequently Asked Questions About Prescription Drug Pricing and Policy, R44832* (Washington, DC: Congressional Research Service, April 24, 2018), 3.

7. Leigh Boerner, "The Complicated Question of Drugs in the Water: Pharmaceuticals— Inescapable in Medicine—Are Increasingly Prevalent in Our Drinking Water. But Is That a Problem?," *NOVA,* May 14, 2014.

8. "AP Finds Prescription Drugs in Drinking Water," *Water and Wastes Digest,* March 10, 2008.

9. Chris V. Thangham, "Pharmaceutical Drugs Found in Water Affects 46 Million Americans," *Digital Journal,* September 11, 2008.

10. Of the 61.3 million women between the ages of 15 and 44, 61.6 percent use some method of contraception. "26.6 Percent of Women Using Contraception Use an Oral Birth Control Pill," National Center for Health Statistics, *Chartbook (2016),* Table 8.

11. Ibid., Table 80.

12. Edward P. Kolodziej and David L. Sedlak, "Rangeland Grazing as a Source of Steroid Hormones to Surface Waters," *Environmental Science & Technology* 41, no. 10 (April 14, 2007): 3514–20.

13. For a reader-friendly explanation of how animal hormones are administered, see Julia Calderone, "The Way Some Meat Producers Fatten Up Cattle Is More Bizarre than You Might Think," *Business Insider,* April 6, 2016.

14. Luke Iwanowicz, email to the author, September 25, 2018.

15. Luke Iwanowicz, author's interview, September 28, 2018.

16. *The Safe Drinking Water Act Amendments of 1996,* §1457 ("Estrogenic Substances Screening Program," 42 U.S.C. §300j-17) provided the EPA with the power to require testing of estrogenic substances. Despite having this authority, the EPA has done little or nothing to test the effect of them. See also the 2010 congressional hearings on endocrine-disrupting chemicals in drinking water, Subcommittee on Energy and the Environment, Serial No. 111–99, February 25, 2010.

17. Luke Iwanowicz, author's interview, September 28, 2018.

18. Luke Iwanowicz et al., "Evidence of Estrogenic Endocrine Disruption in Smallmouth and Largemouth Bass Inhabiting Northeast U.S. National Wildlife Refuge Waters: A Reconnaissance Study," *Ecotoxicology and Environmental Safety* 124 (February 2016): 51–58. See Table 1 for more on the chosen locations.

19. Luke Iwanowicz, author's interview, September 28, 2018.

20. S. Jobling et al., "Wild Intersex Roach (*Rutilus rutilus*) Have Reduced Fertility," *Biology of Reproduction* 67, no. 2 (August 1, 2002): 515–24; and V. S. Blazer et al., "Reproductive Endocrine Disruption in Smallmouth Bass (Micropterus Dolomieu) in the Potomac River Basin: Spatial and Temporal Comparisons of Biological Effects," *Environmental Monitoring and Assessment* 184 (2012): 4309–34.

21. A. M. Vajda, "Reproductive Disruption in Fish Downstream from an Estrogenic Wastewater Effluent," *Environmental Science and Technology* 42, no. 9 (2008): 3407–14.

22. Luke Iwanowicz, author's interview, October 3, 2017.

23. "Great Lakes Facts and Figures," US Environmental Protection Agency, accessed August 10, 2018: https://www.epa.gov/greatlakes/facts-and-figures.

24. For more information on the Great Lakes–St. Lawrence River Basin Water Resources Agreement and Compact, see Peter Annin, *The Great Lakes Water Wars* (Washington, DC: Island Press, 2006).

25. The Great Lakes Region has over 55 million acres of agricultural land under production, consisting of approximately 126,000 farms. US Department of Agriculture, "Great Lakes Region," accessed October 18, 2018: https://www.nrcs.usda.gov/wps/portal/nrcs/detail/national/programs/farmbill/rcpp/?cid=stelprdb1254125; Tom Christensen, Presentation, Associate Chief of Operations, USDA, *Private Lands Voluntary Conservation in the Great Lakes Basin,* US Department of Agriculture (2011). 1,448 wastewater treatment plants discharge into the Great Lakes basin, discharging over 4.8 billion gallons of treated wastewater every day. Antonette Arvai et al., "Protecting Our Great Lakes: Assessing the Effectiveness of Wastewater Treatments for the Removal of Chemicals of Emerging Concern," *Water Quality Research Journal of Canada* 49, no. 1 (2014): 23–31.

26. Diana Aga, author's interview, September 29, 2017.

27. Laura A. Pratt et al., "Antidepressant Use Among Persons Aged 12 and Over: United States, 2011–2014," NCHS Data Brief, no. 283 (Hyattsville, MD: National Center for Health Statistics, August 2017).

28. Professor Aga later explained that, because of the ethical considerations involved, boys before the age of adulthood are not permitted to participate in trials that would require their production of sperm. Nonetheless, in studies of American men, sperm counts have declined over the past several decades, a period that coincides—possibly coincidentally—with the rise of chemicals and pharmaceuticals in drinking water.

29. "Antibiotic/Antimicrobial Resistance (AR/AMR)," Centers for Disease Control and Prevention, National Center for Emerging and Zoonotic Infectious Diseases (NCEZID), accessed October 18, 2018: https://www.cdc.gov/drugresistance/index.html.

30. "WHO's First Global Report on Antibiotic Resistance Reveals Serious, Worldwide Threat to Public Health," press release, World Health Organization, April 30, 2014.

31. Paul Milazzo, email to the author, May 21, 2018.

32. Paola Verlicchi et al., "What Have We Learned from Worldwide Experiences on the Management and Treatment of Hospital Effluent?—An Overview and Discussion on Perspectives," *Science of the Total Environment* 514, (2015): 467–91.

33. "Medical Waste," US Environmental Protection Agency, accessed November 24, 2018: https://www.epa.gov/rcra/medical-waste.

34. Elisabetta Carraro et al., "Hospital Wastewater: Existing Regulations and Current Trends in Management," *Hospital Wastewaters: Characteristics, Management, Treatment and Environmental Risks,* edited by Paola Verlicchi (New York: Springer International Publishing, 2017).

35. National Center for Health Statistics, *Chartbook (2016),* 30.

36. James Baggs et al., "Estimating National Trends in Inpatient Antibiotic Use Among US Hospitals from 2006–2012," *JAMA Internal Medicine* 176, no. 11 (September 2016): 1639–48.

37. Verlicchi et al., "What Have We Learned from Worldwide Experiences on the Management and Treatment of Hospital Effluent?—An Overview and Discussion on Perspectives," 467–91. Those seventeen pharmaceutical classes are: analgesics and anti-inflammatories, anesthetics, anthelmintics, antibiotics, antifungals, antihypertensives, antineoplastics, antiseptics, antivirals, beta-blockers, contrast media, fragrances, hormones, lipid regulators, psychiatric drugs, receptor antagonists, and stimulants.

38. US Department of Health and Human Services, *Guidelines for Environmental Infection Control in Health-Care Facilities* (Atlanta: US Department of Health and Human Services, 2003).

39. Pharmaceutical Input and Elimination from Local Sources (PILLS), *Pharmaceutical Residues in the Aquatic System—A Challenge for the Future* (Gelsenkirchen, Germany: PILLS, September 2012), 4.

40. National Center for Health Statistics, *Chartbook (2016),* Table 89.

41. National Hospice and Palliative Care Organization, *NHPCO Facts and Figures: Hospice Care in America* revised edition (Alexandria, VA: National Hospice and Palliative Care Organization, April 2018), 3–6.

42. Ibid., 2.

43. National Center for Health Statistics, *Chartbook (2016),* Table 80.

44. Heidi Mitchell, "What's the Best Way to Get Rid of Pills You Don't Use?," *Wall Street Journal,* September 26, 2018.

45. Sherri M. Cook et al., "Life Cycle Comparison of Environmental Emissions from Three

Disposal Options for Unused Pharmaceuticals," *Environmental Science & Technology* 46, no. 10 (April 11, 2012): 5535–41.

46. Suzanne Rudzinski, Director, Office of Resource Conservation and Recovery, "Recommendation on the Disposal of Household Pharmaceuticals Collected by Take-Back Events, Mail-Back, and Other Collection Programs," Memorandum to RCRA Division Directors, September 26, 2012.

47. Barbara Whitaker, "Its Notorious Past Unearthed, Dump Loses Landmark Status," *New York Times,* August 29, 2001, A12.

48. Joel Tarr, author's interview, June 12, 2018.

49. US Environmental Protection Agency, *Getting Up to Speed: Ground Water Contamination* (Washington, DC: US Environmental Protection Agency, August 2015), C-4.

50. US Environmental Protection Agency, *Regulatory Impact Analysis for the Proposed Revisions to the Emission Guidelines for Existing Sources and Supplemental Proposed New Source Performance Standards in the Municipal Solid Waste Landfills Sector, EPA-452/R-15-008* (Washington, DC: US Environmental Protection Agency, August 2015), 2–1.

51. The controlling laws here are *Toxic Substances Control Act (TSCA),* 15 U.S.C. ch. 53, subch. I 2601–2629 (1976) and *Resource Conservation and Recovery Act (RCRA),* 42 U.S.C. ch. 82 6901 et seq. (1976). The TSCA provides the EPA with the authority to regulate most chemicals. Regulatory tasks include requiring reporting, record keeping, testing, and, on occasion, restricting certain chemicals. The RCRA provides the EPA with the authority to develop a framework for management of hazardous waste, including chemicals. The RCRA is often described as the "cradle to the grave" law, because it allows the EPA to trace these potentially hazardous chemicals from their first use to their last use or disposal.

52. "Regulations for Municipal Solid Waste Landfills," in "Municipal Solid Waste Landfills," US Environmental Protection Agency, accessed October 19, 2018: https://www.epa.gov /landfills/municipal-solid-waste-landfills. See also *Resource Conservation and Recovery Act (RCRA),* 42 U.S.C. 6901 et seq. (1976).

53. US Environmental Protection Agency, *Advancing Sustainable Materials Management: 2014 Tables and Figures* (Washington, DC: US Environmental Protection Agency, December 2016).

54. US Environmental Protection Agency, *Getting Up to Speed: Ground Water Contamination* (Washington, DC: US Environmental Protection Agency, August 2015), Table 2, C-5.

55. Kim A. O'Connell, "Sorry, Landfill Closed," *Waste360,* July 1, 2001.

56. Rhode Island Department of Health, *Water Quality Protection: Household Hazardous Prod-*

ucts (Providence: Rhode Island Department of Health and University of Rhode Island, March 2004).

57. *Resource Conservation and Recovery Act (RCRA)*. The EPA estimates that there are more than 450,000 properties in the U.S. that have the presence of a hazardous substance that requires remediation. While these sites were not necessarily landfills, they were sites that involved dumping or disposing of hazardous substances. These sites are often referred to as brownfields. "Brownfield Sites," US Environmental Protection Agency, accessed December 19, 2018: https://archive.epa.gov/pesticides/region4/landrevitalization /web/html/brownfieldsites.html.

58. G. Fred Lee and Anne Jones-Lee, *Evaluation of the Potential for a Proposed or Existing Landfill to Pollute Groundwaters* (El Macero, CA: G. Fred Lee & Associates, 1996), 2–3.

59. See, for example, *New York State Public Health Law 201(1), Appendix 75-A, Wastewater Treatment Standards—Residential Onsite Systems* (2016). The twenty-nine pages of septic system criteria include no requirement for ongoing testing for leaks or penalties should leaks occur.

60. "Personal Care Products, Pharmaceuticals, and Hormones Move from Septic Systems to Local Groundwater," US Geological Survey, accessed October 31, 2018: https://toxics .usgs.gov/highlights/2015-06-02_ecs_from_septics.html.

61. State and local regulation of private septic systems varies by location, and regulation is often tied to building permits for new homes—leaving existing, older septic systems unregulated.

62. US Department of Agriculture, Rural Development, HB-1-3555, "Chapter 12: Property and Appraisal Requirements" (Washington, DC: US Department of Agriculture, 2017), 16.

63. P. J. Phillips et al., "Concentrations of Hormones, Pharmaceuticals and Other Micropollutants in Groundwater Affected by Septic Systems in New England and New York," *Science of the Total Environment* 512–13 (April 15, 2015): 43–54.

64. Laurel A. Schaider et al., "Pharmaceuticals, Perfluorosurfactants, and Other Organic Wastewater Compounds in Public Drinking Water Wells in a Shallow Sand and Gravel Aquifer," *Science of the Total Environment* 468–69 (January 15, 2014): 384–87, 391.

65. For a discussion of potable reuse and the presence of contaminants therein, see Steven M. Jones et al., "A Taxonomy of *Chemicals of Emerging Concern* Based on Observed Fate at Water Resource Recovery Facilities," *Chemosphere* 170 (2017): 153–60.

66. Dror Avisar, author's interview, December 26, 2016.

67. Luke Iwanowicz, author's interview, October 3, 2017.

68. Approximately 80 percent of antibiotics used in the U.S. are utilized in meat production. This has led the World Health Organization (WHO) to recommend an end to the routine

use of antibiotics on healthy farm animals. World Health Organization, "Stop Using Antibiotics in Healthy Animals to Prevent the Spread of Antibiotic Resistance," news release (Geneva, Switzerland: World Health Organization, November 7, 2017).

69. Diana Aga, author's interview, September 29, 2017.

70. Dror Avisar, author's interview, January 5, 2017.

71. Dror Avisar, author's interview, December 26, 2016.

FIVE: PLASTIC EVERYWHERE

1. "How much oil is used to make plastic? Frequently Asked Questions," US Energy Information Administration, accessed January 3, 2019: https://www.eia.gov/tools/faqs/faq.php?id=34&t=6.

2. Chemicals Global Industry Almanac, 2017.

3. Agency for Toxic Substances and Disease Registry (ATSDR), *Public Health Statement: Vinyl Chloride, CAS#: 75-01-4* (Atlanta: US Department of Health and Human Services, July 2006).

4. Shanna Swan, author's interview, July 17, 2018. In the game of Whack-A-Mole cited by Dr. Swan, she gave as an example DEHP (di-[2-ethylhexyl] phthalate), a chemical loosely bonded to plastic. Animal studies show that exposure to DEHP can damage the liver, kidneys, lungs, and reproductive system, particularly the developing testes of prenatal and neonatal males. In response to growing complaints and calls to ban it, DINP (di[isononyl] phthalate) and DIDP (di[isodecyl] phthalate) were used as replacements— two substances that have now been associated with the same health concerns.

5. "Bottled Water Becomes Number-One Beverage in the U.S.," press release, Beverage Marketing Corporation, March 10, 2017, accessed October 31, 2018: https://www.prnewswire.com/news-releases/bottled-water-becomes-number-one-beverage-in-the-us-data-from-beverage-marketing-corporation-show-300421385.html.

6. "Bottled Water Advertising," International Bottled Water Association, accessed October 31, 2018: https://www.bottledwater.org/economics/bottled-water-advertising.

7. "Consumers Prefer Bottled Water, Recognize It as a Healthy Choice, and Think It Should Be Available Wherever Drinks are Sold," press release, International Bottled Water Association, December 16, 2017, accessed October 31, 2018: https://www.bottledwater.org/consumers-prefer-bottled-water-recognize-it-healthy-choice-and-think-it-should-be-available-wherever.

8. Proprietary Research Beverage Diary Survey, August 2015.

9. Amy Livingston, "Bottled Water vs. Tap Water—Facts & 4 Reasons to Drink Tap," *Money Crashers,* accessed October 31, 2018: https://www.moneycrashers.com/bottled-water-vs-tap-water-facts/. The author demonstrates that bottled water may be as much as 3,785

times more expensive than tap water. Even taking less expensive bottled water as an example, the disparity is still likely to be more than 1,000-fold greater for bottled water over tap water.

10. Food and Drug Administration, *Requirements for Specific Standardized Beverages, Bottled Water, 21 CFR 165.110.*

11. Erik D. Olson, *Bottled Water: Pure Drink or Pure Hype?* (Washington, DC: Natural Resources Defense Council, February 1999, Updated Commentary, September 2, 2010), 23–36. See also Malwina Diduch et al., "Chemical Quality of Bottled Waters: A Review," *Journal of Food Science* 76, no. 9 (November 9, 2011): R178–R196.

12. Gary Hemphill, Managing Director of Research, Beverage Marketing Corporation, email to the author, July 2, 2018.

13. Sales Statistics are from "Consumers Reaffirm Bottled Water Is America's Favorite Drink," press release, International Bottled Water Association, May 31, 2018, accessed November 1, 2018: https://www.bottledwater.org/consumers-reaffirm-bottled-water -america's-favorite-drink.

14. Adrianna Quintero, "Bottled Water: Still Pure Hype," Natural Resources Defense Council, September 2, 2010.

15. Nelson Switzer, author's interview, November 20, 2017.

16. See Food and Drug Administration, *Requirements for Specific Standardized Beverages, Bottled Water, 21 CFR 165.110.*

17. "Beverages: Bottled Water: Final Rule," 60 Federal Register 57,076, at 57,120, November 13, 1995: "The agency [FDA] advises that the act only applies to food that is in, or is intended to be shipped in, interstate commerce. . . . FDA encourages States to apply the Federal standard to both interstate and intrastate commerce to eliminate two levels of regulation and to avoid undue logistical burdens."

18. Quintero, "Bottled Water: Still Pure Hype."

19. Drinking Water Research Foundation, *Bottled Water and Tap Water: Just the Facts—A Comparison of Regulatory Requirements for Quality and Monitoring of Drinking Water in the United States* (Alexandria, VA: Drinking Water Research Foundation, March 2014), 7.

20. "Consumers Prefer Bottled Water, Recognize It as a Healthy Choice, and Think It Should Be Available Wherever Drinks are Sold," press release, International Bottled Water Association, December 16, 2017, accessed October 31, 2018: https://www.bottled water.org/consumers-prefer-bottled-water-recognize-it-healthy-choice-and-think-it -should-be-available-wherever.

21. See Matthew Boesler, "You Are Paying 300 Times More for Bottled Water than Tap Water," *Slate,* July 12, 2013; and G. E. Miller, "The TRUE Cost of Bottled Water vs. Tap Water (& Comparative Purity & Taste Test Results)," *20 Something Finance,* December 28, 2018.

22. Oliver Balch, "The Madness of Drinking Bottled Water Shipped Halfway Round the World," *The Guardian,* July 9, 2015.

23. "FAQ: How is DASANI Made?," Dasani, accessed December 30, 2018: https://www.dasani.com/faq/; "FAQ: How is Aquafina Purified?," Aquafina, accessed December 30, 2018: https://www.aquafina.com/en-US/faq.html.

24. Kevin Miller, "Maine's Top Court Upholds Sale of Fryeburg Water to Poland Spring," *Portland Press Herald,* May 13, 2016.

25. Lawrence J. Speer, "Nestlé Relaunches Perrier in Plastic Bottles," *Ad Age,* May 1, 2001.

26. Roland Geyer et al., "Production, Use, and Fate of all Plastics Ever Made," *Science Advances* 3 (July 2017): 1–5.

27. Radoslaw Czernych et al., "Characterization of Estrogenic and Androgenic Activity of Phthalates by the XenoScreen YES/YAS in Vitro Assay," *Environmental Toxicology and Pharmacology* 53 (2017): 95–104.

28. Qiong Luo et al., "Migration and Potential Risk of Trace Phthalates in Bottled Water: A Global Situation," *Water Research* 147 (2018): 362–72.

29. Gary Hemphill, Managing Director of Research, Beverage Marketing Corporation, email to the author, July 2, 2018.

30. Martin Wagner et al., "Identification of Putative Steroid Receptor Antagonists in Bottled Water: Combining Bioassays and High-Resolution Mass Spectrometry," *PLoS ONE* 8, no. 8 (August 2013): e72472.

31. Martin Wagner, email to the author, July 29, 2018.

32. Martin Wagner, author's interview, July 26, 2018.

33. Jane Houlihan et al., "Timeline: BPA from Invention to Phase-Out," *Environmental Working Group*, April 22, 2008.

34. Center for the Evaluation of Risks to Human Reproduction, *Monograph on the Potential Human Reproductive and Developmental Effects of Bisphenol A, NIH Publication No. 08–5994* (Research Triangle Park, NC: Center for the Evaluation of Risks to Human Reproduction, National Toxicology Program, September 2008).

35. Johanna R. Rochester, "Bisphenol A and Human Health: A Review of the Literature," *Reproductive Toxicology* 42 (December 2013): 132–55.

36. National Conference of State Legislatures (NCSL), NCSL Policy Update: State Restrictions on Bisphenol A (BPA) in Consumer Products, February 2015, accessed December 30, 2018: http://www.ncsl.org/research/environment-and-natural-resources/policy-update-on-state-restrictions-on-bisphenol-a.aspx.

37. Jenna Bilbrey, "BPA-Free Plastic Containers May Be Just as Hazardous," *Scientific American,* August 11, 2014; and Robert F. Service, "BPA Substitutes May Be Just as Bad as the Popular Consumer Plastic," *Science,* September 13, 2018.

38. Shanna Swan, author's interview, July 17, 2018.

39. "Medical Management Guidelines for Vinyl Chloride," Centers for Disease Control and prevention, Agency for Toxic Substances and Disease Registry (ATSDR), October 21, 2014, accessed December 30, 2018: https://www.atsdr.cdc.gov/MMG/MMG .asp?id=278&tid=84.

40. Andrew Whelton, author's interview, December 9, 2018.

41. Polyethylene pipes used to transport drinking water have also become a source of concern. After installation of them by Cambridge, Massachusetts, a decision was made to begin testing them to see if chemicals leaching from them caused harm. See Sue Reinert, "Lingering Fear About Plastic-Lined Water Pipes Encourages City to Take the Lead on Safety Tests," *Cambridge Day,* December 20, 2018

42. Andrew J. Whelton, Letter to the Editor, "Comments on 'PEX and PP Water Pipes: Assimilable Carbon, Chemicals, and Odors,'" *Journal AWWA* 108, no. 8 (August 2016): 12–13.

43. Andrew J. Whelton, "Why Is Our Plumbing Harming Us?," Presentation at Dawn or Doom Technology Conference, Purdue University (October 4, 2016), 20.

44. Andrew Whelton, author's interview, December 9, 2018.

45. David Stradling and Richard Stradling, "Perceptions of the Burning River: Deindustrialization and Cleveland's Cuyahoga River," *Environmental History* 13, no. 3 (July 1, 2008): 515–35.

46. PlasticsEurope, Association of Plastics Manufacturers, *Plastics—The Facts 2017: An Analysis of European Plastics Production, Demand and Waste Data* (Brussels, Belgium: PlasticsEurope, 2018), 16.

47. Martin Wagner, author's interview, July 26, 2018.

48. Jenna R. Jambeck et al., "Plastic Waste Inputs from Land into the Ocean," *Science* 347, no. 6223 (February 13, 2015): 768–71.

49. Julia Reisser et al., "Marine Plastic Pollution in Waters Around Australia: Characteristics, Concentrations, and Pathways," *PLoS ONE* 8, no. 11 (November 2013): e80466.

50. *Microbead-Free Waters Act of 2015,* §331 21 U.S.C. (2015).

51. Martin Wagner and Scott Lambert, *Freshwater Microplastics: Emerging Environmental Contaminants?* (Cham, Switzerland: Springer Nature, 2018), 28.

52. Mary Kosuth et al., "Anthropogenic Contamination of Tap Water, Beer, and Sea Salt," *PLoS ONE* 13, no. 4 (April 2018): e0194970.

53. Darena Schymanski et al., "Analysis of Microplastics in Water by Micro-Raman Spectroscopy: Release of Plastic Particles from Different Packaging into Mineral Water," *Water Research* 129 (November 2017): 154–62.

54. Kosuth, et al., "Anthropogenic Contamination of Tap Water, Beer, and Sea Salt."

55. Martin Wagner, email to the author, December 28, 2018.

56. Wagner and Lambert, *Freshwater Microplastics: Emerging Environmental Contaminants?*, 154.

57. Martin Wagner, author's interview, July 26, 2018.

58. See "Comments from the Natural Resources Defense Council on Proposed Procedures for Chemical Risk Evaluation Under the Amended Toxic Substances Control Act," Submitted to Docket EPA-HQ-OPPT-2016-0654, March 20, 2017.

59. Veena Singla, author's interview, June 18, 2018.

60. Veena Singla, author's interview, June 15, 2018.

SIX: ONE CITY OF MANY: FLINT AND LEAD IN AMERICA'S DRINKING WATER

1. "Quick Facts: Flint, Michigan," US Census Bureau, accessed October 14, 2018: https://www.census.gov/quickfacts/flintcitymichigan.

2. Two books about the Flint water crisis ably tell the story. Mona Hanna-Attisha, *What the Eyes Don't See: A Story of Crisis, Resistance, and Hope in an American City* (New York: One World, 2018), is the more personal of the books. Dr. Hanna-Attisha, a pediatrician at a Flint hospital, helped to raise awareness of the crisis. She movingly records the failure of government to respond promptly to an unfolding medical emergency. Anna Clark's book, *The Poisoned City: Flint's Water and the American Urban Tragedy* (New York: Metropolitan Books/Henry Holt, 2018), is a journalist's account of the Flint story. It not only helps to explain how the crisis came to be, it also rounds out the picture of how a city's infrastructure came to fail the citizens it was built to serve.

3. Hanna-Attisha, *What the Eyes Don't See: A Story of Crisis, Resistance, and Hope in an American City*, 226.

4. US Environmental Protection Agency, *Lead and Copper Rule Revisions White Paper* (Washington, DC: US Environmental Protection Agency, Office of Water, October 2016), 5.

5. Bruce P. Lanphear et al., "Low-Level Lead Exposure and Mortality in US Adults: A Population-Based Cohort Study," *The Lancet* 3, no. 4 (March 12, 2018): E177–84.

6. Government Accountability Office, *Drinking Water: Approaches for Identifying Lead Service Lines Should be Shared with All States, GAO-18-620* (Washington, DC: Government Acscountability Office, 2018), 10.

7. Mike Schock, author's interview, October 17, 2018.

8. Horsley Whitten Group, Inc. and W. K. Kellogg Foundation, *Managing Lead in Drinking Water at Schools and Early Childhood Facilities* (Battle Creek, MI: W. K. Kellogg Foundation, February 2016), 1–4. For representative news reports about lead in schools, see Kate Galbraith, "Alarm over Lead Found in Drinking Water at US Schools," *The Guard-*

ian, March 1, 2016; and Brady Dennis, "Facing Pressure, More Schools Scramble to Confront Dangers of Lead in Water," *Washington Post,* April 30, 2017.

9. *ACORN v. Edwards,* 81 F.3d 1387 (5th Cir. 1996).

10. *Water Infrastructure Improvements for the Nation Act,* P.L. 114–322, title II, §2107(a), December 16, 2016, 130 Stat. 1727.

11. Yanna Lambrinidou et al., "Failing Our Children: Lead in US School Drinking Water," *New Solutions* 20, no. 1 (2010): 41.

12. Erik Olson and Kristi Pullen Fedinick, *What's in Your Water? Flint and Beyond: Analysis of EPA Data Reveals Widespread Lead Crisis Potentially Affecting Millions of Americans* (Washington, DC: Natural Resources Defense Council, 2016).

13. Martin V. Melosi, *Precious Commodity: Providing Water for America's Cities* (Pittsburgh: University of Pittsburgh Press, 2011), 57–77.

14. James Proctor, author's interview, November 9, 2018.

15. Werner Troesken, *The Great Lead Water Pipe Disaster* (Cambridge: MIT Press, 2006), 10–12.

16. Mike Schock, author's interview, October 17, 2018.

17. AWWA Research Foundation, *Contribution of Service Line and Plumbing Fixtures to Lead and Copper Rule Compliance Issues* (Denver: AWWA Research Foundation, 2008), 56.

18. Randolph K. Byers and Elizabeth E. Lord, "Late Effects of Lead Poisoning on Mental Development," *Journal of Diseases of Children* 66, no. 5 (1943): 471–94.

19. Herbert L. Needleman and David Bellinger, "The Health Effect of Low Level Exposure to Lead," *Annual Review of Public Health* 12, no. 111-40 (1991): 123.

20. Herbert Needleman et al., "Bone Lead Levels in Adjudicated Delinquents: A Case Control Study," *Neurotoxicology & Teratology* 24, no. 6 (November–December 2002): 711–17.

21. Karen Clay et al., *Lead Pipes and Child Mortality, Working Paper 12603,* National Bureau of Economic Research (Cambridge, MA: National Bureau of Economic Research, October 2006), 5–6.

22. Troesken, *The Great Lead Water Pipe Disaster,* 123–40.

23. For a history of anticorrosives, see Xiaotao Guan, "Impact of Zinc Orthophosphate Inhibitor on Distribution System Water Quality," PhD diss., Department of Civil and Environmental Engineering in the College of Engineering and Computer Science (Orlando: University of Central Florida, 2007).

24. Lauren W. Wasserstrom et al., "Scale Formation Under Blended Phosphate Treatment for a Utility with Lead Pipes," *Journal AWWA* 109, no. 11 (November 2017): E464.

25. The EPA's 1991 Lead and Copper Rule lowered the safe limit of lead from 50 parts per billion down to 15 parts per billion. "Control of Lead and Copper," 40 CFR Part 141 Subpart I.

26. Mike Schock, author's interview, October 17, 2018.

27. Peter C. Grevatt, Director, Office of Ground Water and Drinking Water, "Clarification of Recommended Tap Sampling Procedures for Purposes of the Lead and Copper Rule," Memorandum to Water Division Directors, US Environmental Protection Agency, February 29, 2016.

28. Mike Schock, email to the author, November 3, 2018.

29. US Environmental Protection Agency, *Lead and Copper Rule Monitoring and Reporting Guidance for Public Water Systems, EPA 816-R-10-004* (Washington, DC: US Environmental Protection Agency, revised March 2010), 15–22.

30. "Control of Lead and Copper," 40 CFR Part 141 Subpart I, §141.8(c).

31. Although the interviewee here was speaking more generally, for a recent example, see Michael Hawthorne and Jennifer Smith Richards, "Chicago Often Tests Water for Lead in Homes Where Risk is Low," *Chicago Tribune,* February 26, 2016.

32. Oliver Milman and Jessica Glenza, "At Least 33 US Cities Used Water Testing 'Cheats' over Lead Concerns," *The Guardian,* June 2, 2016.

33. Oliver Milman, "US Authorities Distorting Tests to Downplay Lead Content of Water," *The Guardian,* January 22, 2016.

34. To be fair, there are some noteworthy exceptions. Cincinnati is known for its forward-looking drinking water utility. The utility there takes lead samples more often than required and it goes to great pains to verify that the houses selected for sampling are of a vintage that might have a lead service line or other lead problem.

35. Adele Peters, "This Activist Is Still Fighting to Get Flint Clean Water," *Fast Company,* May 1, 2018.

36. Miguel Del Toral, Regulations Manager, Ground Water and Drinking Water Branch, US Environmental Protection Agency, "High Lead Levels in Flint, Michigan—Interim Report," Memorandum to Thomas Poy, Chief, Office of Ground Water and Drinking Water, US Environmental Protection Agency, June 24, 2015.

37. *Concerned Pastors for Social Action, et al. v. Khouri, et al.,* Case No. 2:16-cv-10277, US District Court, Eastern District of Michigan; and *Jan Burgess, et al., v. United States of America,* Case No. 2:17-cv-10291, US District Court, Eastern District of Michigan.

38. Settlement Agreement, *Concerned Pastors for Social Action, et al. v. Khouri, et al., Case No. 2:16-cv-10277,* US District Court, Eastern District of Michigan, March 23, 2017.

39. Virginia Gewin, "Turning Point: Activist Engineer," *Nature* 537 (September 14, 2016): 439.

40. DC Water, "WASA Board Approves Plan to Replace All D.C. Lead Service Lines," press release (Washington, DC: DC Water, July 1, 2004).

41. Marc Edwards, author's interview, May 4, 2018.

42. Centers for Disease Control and Prevention, "Blood Lead Levels in Residents of Homes with Elevated Lead in Tap Water—District of Columbia, 2004," *MMWR Weekly* 53, no. 12 (April 2, 2004): 268–70.

43. Marc Edwards, email to the author, August 14, 2018.

44. Subcommittee on Investigations and Oversight of the Committee on Science and Technology, US House of Representatives, *A Public Health Tragedy: How Flawed CDC Data and Faulty Assumptions Endangered Children's Health in the Nation's Capital,* Report to Subcommittee Chairman Brad Miller, May 20, 2010.

45. Centers for Disease Control and Prevention, "Notice to Readers: Limitations Inherent to a Cross-Sectional Assessment of Blood Lead Levels Among Persons Living in Homes with High Levels of Lead in Drinking Water," *MMWR Weekly* 59, no. 24 (June 25, 2010): 751.

46. Marc Edwards, email to the author, August 14, 2018.

47. Marc Edwards, author's interview, May 4, 2018.

48. LeadFreeNYC, *A Roadmap to Eliminating Childhood Lead Exposure* (New York: Lead-FreeNYC, Mayor's Office of Operations Task Force, 2019), 24.

49. Bill de Blasio, author's interview, February 17, 2019.

50. Hank Habicht, author's interview, October 26, 2018.

SEVEN: THE WATER INDUSTRY

1. Don D. Ratnayaka et al., *Twort's Water Supply,* 6th edition (Oxford, UK: Elsevier, 2009), 39. Also, Martin Melosi, author's interview, October 23, 2018.

2. In addition to the 51,535 water utilities, and contributing even less coherence to this bloated system, there are also more than 100,000 "noncommunity water systems," such as schools, hospitals, and campgrounds that have their own water supply that is not—but could be—hooked up to a local water utility. "Background on Drinking Water Standards in the Safe Drinking Water Act (SDWA)," US Environmental Protection Agency, accessed January 7, 2019: https://www.epa.gov/dwstandardsregulations /background-drinking-water-standards-safe-drinking-water-act-sdwa.

3. American Water Works Association (AWWA), *2015 AWWA State of the Water Industry Report* (Denver: American Water Works Association, 2015), 11.

4. National Research Council, *Privatization of Water Services in the United States: An Assessment of Issues and Experience* (Washington, DC: National Academies Press, 2002), 30–34.

5. Larry Lai, *Adopting County Policies Which Limit Public Water System Sprawl and Promote Small System Consolidation* (Los Angeles: University of California, Los Angeles, Luskin School of Public Affairs, May 2017), 15.

6. Felicia Marcus, author's interview, September 21, 2018.

7. Mike Keegan, author's interview, August 16, 2018.

8. American Water Works Association (AWWA), *2015 State of the Water Industry Report.*

9. US Environmental Protection Agency, *Drinking Water: EPA Needs to Take Additional Steps to Ensure Small Community Water Systems Designated as Serious Violators Achieve Compliance, Report No. 16-P-0108* (Washington, DC: US Environmental Protection Agency, March 22, 2016); Maura Allaire et al., "National Trends in Drinking Water Quality Violations," *PNAS* 115, no. 9 (February 27, 2018): 2078–83; and Daniel Irvin, "Trends in EPA Violations in Water Systems," UNC School of Government, February 8, 2017.

10. Kristi Pullen Fedinick et al., *Threats on Tap: Widespread Violations Highlight Need for Investment in Water Infrastructure and Protections* (Washington, DC: Natural Resources Defense Council, May 2017), 4.

11. *Safe Drinking Water Act Amendments of 1996,* 42 U.S.C. 300f–300j, as amended by P.L. 104–182, "Unregulated Contaminants," §1445 (42 U.S.C. 300j-4).

12. US Environmental Protection Agency, *Variances and Exemptions: A Quick Reference Guide, EPA 816-F-04-005* (Washington, DC: US Environmental Protection Agency, Office of Water, September 2004).

13. Kenneth Johnson, *Demographic Trends in Rural and Small Town America* (Durham: University of New Hampshire, Carsey Institute, 2006), 27–31.

14. Joseph Kane and Adie Tomer, *Renewing the Water Workplace: Improving Water Infrastructure and Creating a Pipeline to Opportunity* (Washington, DC: Metropolitan Policy Program at Brookings, June 2018), 17.

15. Ibid., 5.

16. Ibid., 10.

17. Steve Fletcher, National Rural Water Association, Witness Statement, "Drinking Water System Improvement Act of 2017," US House of Representatives, Subcommittee on the Environment, May 19, 2019.

18. Ratnayaka et al., *Twort's Water Supply,* 39.

19. National Research Council, *Privatization of Water Services in the United States: An Assessment of Issues and Experience,* 37–38.

20. Martin V. Melosi, *Precious Commodity: Providing Water for America's Cities* (Pittsburgh: University of Pittsburgh Press, 2011), 58.

21. Although not as comprehensive as in the United Kingdom, Kentucky is an example of a slow-moving consolidation process. In 1979, there were approximately two thousand water utilities. There are about four hundred today. See CoBank, *Rural Infrastructure Briefings: When Rural Water Systems Combine* (Greenwood Village, CO: CoBank ACB, October 2017).

22. "Contact Details—Your Water Company," Ofwat, accessed December 31, 2018: https://www.ofwat.gov.uk/households/your-water-company/map/.

23. Chief Inspector of Drinking Water, *Drinking Water Quality in England: The Position After 25 Years of Regulation* (London: Drinking Water Inspectorate, 2015); Sara Priestley and Thomas Rutherford, "Water Bills—Affordability and Support for Household Customers," Briefing Paper CBP06596 (London: House of Commons Library, August 2016); "Water Companies to Cut Bills in England and Wales," BBC News, September 3, 2018.

24. Office of Water Services (Ofwat), *The Development of the Water Industry in England and Wales* (Birmingham, UK: Ofwat, 2006), 1–3, 35–40, 47, 53, 77–81, 87–89.

25. To be sure, the AWWA isn't the only organization that speaks to Congress and federal agencies about drinking water issues from the perspective of the drinking water industry. Among others, the Association of Metropolitan Water Agencies (the largest publicly owned water utilities) and the National Association of Water Companies (private drinking water service providers) also play a part. There are also important organizations focused primarily on wastewater issues that may overlap with drinking water such as the National Association of Clean Water Agencies and the Water Environment Federation. In addition, the American Society of Civil Engineers (ASCE) has a large global membership among which many of its civil engineer members work in water infrastructure and in water-related fields. ASCE also speaks with Congress and federal agencies about issues of concern to its members.

26. In explaining how the organization straddles these two potentially adverse positions, the AWWA's director of communications writes: "It's true that AWWA considers the perspective of utilities, and it's also true that public health is a core value. We advocate for sound science that helps assure each dollar is spent in a way that best advances public health protection." Greg Kail, email to the author, November 13, 2018.

27. David LaFrance, author's interview, August 20, 2018.

28. G. Tracy Mehan III, author's interview, August 1, 2018.

29. Greg Kail, email to the author, November 13, 2018.

30. American Water Works Association, *Dawn of the Replacement Era: Reinvesting in Drinking Water Infrastructure* (Denver: American Water Works Association, May 2001), 6. Although nothing more than a curiosity today, in the era before cast iron pipes, some communities used wood pipes fitted together like a wooden barrel and then lashed closed with wire. In a handful of remote places, these wooden pipes are still in use. See Michael Cooper, "Aging of Water Mains Is Becoming Hard to Ignore," *New York Times,* April 17, 2009.

31. Peter Williams, author's interview, September 28, 2018.

32. American Society of Civil Engineers (ASCE), *2017 Infrastructure Report Card: A Comprehensive Assessment of America's Infrastructure* (Reston, VA: American Society of Civil Engineers, 2017), 36–37.

33. In a report on water loss, 246 utilities reported 29.4 billion gallons of water lost at a cost of $151 million in lost fees. Extrapolating those figures, a national water loss of two trillion gallons yields lost revenue of $10.2 billion. Even if lower numbers were to be used in this extrapolation, the amount lost nationally is, to quote that report, "staggering." American Water Works Association, *The State of Water Loss Control in Drinking Water Utilities,* American Water Works Association, White Paper (Denver: American Water Works Association, 2016), 6.

34. American Society of Civil Engineers (ASCE), *2017 Infrastructure Report Card.*

35. Steven Folkman, "Water Main Break Rates in the USA and Canada: A Comprehensive Study," *Mechanical and Aerospace Engineering Faculty Publications* (March 2018), Paper 174.

36. The $1 trillion estimate provided by the American Water Works Association is higher than those of the EPA, the Congressional Budget Office, and the Water Infrastructure Network because it also includes the cost of expanding pipe networks to meet growing population needs. Since it is realistic to assume that population will continue to expand, the AWWA scenario seems most likely. US Environmental Protection Agency, *Drinking Water Infrastructure Needs Survey and Assessment, Sixth Report to Congress, EPA 816-K-17-002* (Washington, DC: US Environmental Protection Agency, March 2018), 20.

37. American Water Works Association, *Buried No Longer: Confronting America's Water Infrastructure Challenge* (Denver: American Water Works Association, February 27, 2012), 10.

38. American Water Works Association, *Dawn of the Replacement Era,* 6.

39. James Proctor, author's interview, November 9, 2018.

40. After a few cities and towns began assessing fees for firefighting services, several states banned municipalities from doing so. See Sarah Netter, "Fire Departments Charge for Service, Asking Accident Victims to Pay Up," *ABC News,* February 4, 2010.

41. Brett Walton, "Infographic: Average U.S. Household Water Use and Bills," *Circle of Blue,* May 18, 2016. AWWA CEO David LaFrance suggests an explanation for this disparity by comparing the cost of upkeep for Boston's aged water infrastructure, the large transportation cost for San Francisco's water, and the rapid population growth in Phoenix, where the fixed costs have a larger base among which it is allocated. David LaFrance, email to the author, November 13, 2018.

42. Ted Gregory et al., "The Water Drain: Same Lake, Unequal Rates," *Chicago Tribune,* October 25, 2017.

43. For a commonsense approach to water fees, see "Policy Statement: Financing, Accounting, and Rates," American Water Works Association, revised June 7, 2015, ac-

cessed December 30, 2018: https://www.awwa.org/Policy-Advocacy/AWWA-Policy
-Statements/Financing-Accounting-and-Rates.

44. Jay van Santen, "The End Is Here: Cable's Media Dominance," *Seeking Alpha,* September 12, 2017.

45. Janice Beecher, "Trends in Consumer Expenditures and Prices for Public Utilities (2018)," Institute of Public Utilities, Michigan State University (June 2, 2018).

46. It is easy to issue grand proclamations while leaving the hard work of devising the solution to others. But here, as challenging as the details will be to develop, sell to the stakeholders, and implement, the greatest challenge is to get broad agreement that there is a problem and that consolidation should be the first step to a solution.

EIGHT: PUSHING THE EPA TO DO MORE

1. Erik Olson, author's interview, October 19, 2018.

2. Jonathan Nichols, author's interview, October 11, 2018.

3. Peter Bower, author's interview, October 17, 2018.

4. National Science Teachers Association, *Programs in Environmental Education* (Washington, DC: National Science Teachers Association, 1970).

5. Erik Olson, author's interview, January 31, 2018.

6. "Environmental and Land Use Law," University of Virginia School of Law, accessed October 12, 2018: https://www.law.virginia.edu/academics/program/environmental -and-land-use-law.

7. Erik D. Olson, "The Quiet Shift of Power: Office of Management and Budget Supervision of Environmental Protection Agency Rulemaking Under Executive Order 12,291," *Virginia Journal of Natural Resources Law* 4, no. 1 (1984).

8. *Natural Resources Defense Council v. United States Department of Defense,* 442 F.Supp.2d 857 (2006). Also see Erik Olson and Jennifer Sass, "White House and Pentagon Bias National Academy Perchlorate Report," Natural Resources Defense Council, January 10, 2005.

9. National Wildlife Federation, *Danger on Tap: The Government's Failure to Enforce the Federal Safe Drinking Water Act, FY 1988 Update* (Washington, DC: National Wildlife Federation, Environmental Quality Division, 1989); and National Wildlife Federation, *Danger on Tap: State by State Data Tables* (Washington, DC: National Wildlife Federation, Environmental Quality Division, Washington, DC, 2008).

10. John N. Adams and Patricia Adams, *Force for Nature: The Story of NRDC and the Fight to Save Our Planet* (San Francisco: Chronicle Books, 2010), 82–83.

11. J. Gustave Speth, *Angels by the River* (White River Junction, VT: Chelsea Green Publishing, 2014), 125–28.

12. John Adams, author's interview, June 8, 2018.

13. Gus Speth, author's interview, July 27, 2018.

14. The NRDC's far-from-routine effort to get tax-exempt status is told in some detail in Adams and Adams, *Force for Nature: The Story of NRDC and the Fight to Save Our Planet,* 22–30.

15. John Adams, author's interview, June 9, 2018.

16. Erik D. Olson, *Think Before You Drink: The Failure of the Nation's Drinking Water System to Protect Public Health* (Washington, DC: Natural Resources Defense Council, September 1993), i–viii. See also *Think Before You Drink: 1992–1993 Update* (July 1994).

17. Olson and the NRDC regularly issued drinking water–themed reports that discussed both policy and science in support of stronger drinking water laws, regulation, and enforcement. In the period before the 1996 Amendments, in addition to *Think Before You Drink* and its *Update,* other reports included *Victorian Water Treatment Enters the 21st Century: Public Health Threats from Water Utilities' Ancient Treatment and Distribution Systems* (March 1994), *The Dirty Little Secret About Our Drinking Water* (February 1995), and *You Are What You Drink: Cryptosporidium and Other Contaminants Found in the Water Served to Millions of Americans* (June 1995). The NRDC also jointly prepared and issued *Just Add Water* with the Environmental Working Group.

18. Subcommittee on Arsenic in Drinking Water, Committee on Toxicology, Board on Environmental Studies and Toxicology, Commission on Life Sciences, National Research Council, *Arsenic in Drinking Water* (Washington, DC: National Academy Press, 1999), 83–124.

19. Paul Mushak et al., *Arsenic and Old Laws: Arsenic Occurrence in Drinking Water, Its Health Effects, and the EPA's Outdated Tap Water Standard* (Washington, DC: Natural Resources Defense Council, 2000), 15–16.

20. US Environmental Protection Agency, *Drinking Water Standard for Arsenic, EPA 815-F-00-015* (Washington, DC: US Environmental Protection Agency, January 2001).

21. Steven H. Lamm et al., "Arsenic Cancer Risk Confounder in Southwest Taiwan Data Set," *Environmental Health Perspectives* 114, no. 7 (July 2006): 1077–82.

22. Subcommittee on Arsenic in Drinking Water, *Arsenic in Drinking Water,* 10–12.

23. Timothy Egan, "In New Mexico, Debate over Arsenic Strikes Home," *New York Times,* April 14, 2001, A1.

24. When the arsenic standard was lowered in 2001, water engineers in Albuquerque blended in low- or no-arsenic water from other wells or from a newly constructed $6.3 million water treatment plant into the municipal water supply. This produced water below the new, lowered EPA standard, and at a cost of 3 percent of the $200 million earlier claimed by the local water utility and repeated by Senator Domenici. Not only wasn't Albuquerque obliged to spend $200 million to get safer water for its citizens, it didn't even spend $6.3 million, as the treatment plant was built with financial assistance from the federal

government. See "Your Drinking Water: Arsenic Compliance & Health Effects," Albuquerque Bernalillo County Water Utility Authority, accessed November 11, 2018: http://www.abcwua.org/Arsenic_Compliance_and_Health_Effects.aspx.

25. Senate Amendment 2964 to HR 5679, 102nd Congress, September 9, 1992.

26. Erik Olson, author's interview, April 13, 2018.

27. Mushak et al., *Arsenic and Old Laws: Arsenic Occurrence in Drinking Water, Its Health Effects, and the EPA's Outdated Tap Water Standard.*

28. "NRDC Sues to Force White House to Release New EPA Standard for Arsenic Levels in Tap Water," press release, Natural Resources Defense Council, May 10, 2000.

29. Frank Bove et al., "Drinking Water Contaminants and Adverse Pregnancy Outcomes: A Review," *Environmental Health Perspectives* 110, no. 1 (February 2002), 61–74.

30. Erik Olson, author's interview, June 20, 2018.

31. Phaedra S. Corso et al., "Costs of Illness in the 1993 Waterborne Cryptosporidium Outbreak, Milwaukee, Wisconsin," *Emerging Infectious Diseases* 9, no. 4 (April 2003): 426–31.

32. Full protection against Legionella would require not just improved disinfection and filtration at the water treatment plant, but also better management of the pipes that distribute the water. Once Legionella gets into the pipes, it can be harbored and grow there. See Stephen A. Hubbs, "Addressing Legionella: Public Health Enemy #1 in US Water Systems," Water Quality and Health Council, August 29, 2014.

33. Environmental Working Group, *Pesticides in Baby Food* (Washington, DC: Environmental Working Group, July 1, 1995). In the twenty years following the passage of the *Food Quality Protection Act*, the passage of which was aided by the release of *Pesticides in Baby Food,* the volume of pesticides found in baby food dropped significantly. See Sonya Lunder, "In 20 Years, Pesticides in Baby Food Drop Dramatically," Environmental Working Group, August 3, 2016.

34. Environmental Working Group, *Weed Killers by the Glass* (Washington, DC: Environmental Working Group, September 1, 1995).

35. Ken Cook, author's interviews, June 18, 26, and 29, 2018.

36. David Zwick and Marcy Benstock, *Water Wasteland* (New York: Grossman Publishers, 1971).

37. Lynn Thorp, author's interview, June 21, 2018.

38. Clean Water Action, *Celebrating the Life & Legacy of David Zwick,* Memorial Booklet, June 7, 2018.

39. Maureo Fernández y Mora, author's interview, January 4, 2019.

40. Clean Water Action, *Protecting Groundwater from the Ground Up, White Paper.*

41. Thomas Harter et al., *Addressing Nitrate in California's Drinking Water* (Davis: Center for Watershed Sciences, University of California, Davis, March 2012).

42. Jennifer Clary, author's interview, October 1, 2018.

43. Lynn Thorp, author's interview, June 19, 2018

44. David Mebane, "Raw sewage polluting Little Bighorn," *Big Horn County News*, 1993, 1.

45. Montana State University, *Crow Reservation—Montana Poverty Report Card* (Bozeman, MT: Montana State University, August 2017).

46. John Doyle, author's interview, January 31, 2019.

47. Michele Roberts, author's interview, February 1, 2019.

48. "Drinking Water Requirements for States and Public Water Systems: Surface Water Treatment Rules," US Environmental Protection Agency, accessed December 30, 2018: https://www.epa.gov/dwreginfo/surface-water-treatment-rules.

49. New York State Department of Health, US Environmental Protection Agency, "New York City Filtration Avoidance Determination, 2017 Surface Water Treatment Rule Determination for New York City's Catskill/Delaware Water Supply System," December 2017.

50. Eric Goldstein, author's interview, April 24, 2018.

51. Ibid.

NINE: WHY CAN'T WE ALL HAVE WATER LIKE ORANGE COUNTY?

1. Allison Lassiter, *Sustainable Water: Challenges and Solutions from California* (Oakland: University of California Press, 2015), 226–28.

2. National Research Council, *Use of Reclaimed Water and Sludge in Food Crop Production* (Washington, DC: National Academies Press, 1996), 142–43.

3. *Federal Water Pollution Control Act (Clean Water Act),* 33 USC §§1251–1387 (1972).

4. For a detailed history of southern California's early water projects, see Marc Reisner, *Cadillac Desert: The American West and Its Disappearing Water* (New York: Penguin, 1986), Chapter 2.

5. The Colorado River and its tributaries provide water for nearly 40 million people and 5.5 million acres of irrigated farm land. US Bureau of Reclamation, *Colorado River Basin Water Supply and Demand Study, Executive Summary* (US Department of the Interior, December 2012), 3.

6. Forest Tennant, author's interview, February 10, 2018.

7. Patricia Tennyson, author's interview, December 20, 2017.

8. City of San Diego, *Annual Drinking Water Quality Report* (2016), 3.

9. Marti Emerald, author's interview, December 22, 2017.

10. Devon Lantry, "What's in the Water? What's in a Word?," *Waterkeeper Alliance* 12, no. 1 (Winter 2016).

11. Kenneth Chang, "NEXT L.A.: The Water Cycle Gets Recycled: The East Valley Water Project Plans to Reuse Waste Water After Letting It Percolate Through the Soil for Five Years," *Los Angeles Times,* December 5, 1995.

12. Gerald A. Silver, author's interview, December 19, 2017.

13. Rick Orlov, "'Toilet to Tap' Flap Bubbles Up," *Los Angeles Daily News,* June 6, 2000.

14. Gerald A. Silver, author's interview, December 19, 2017.

15. D. J. Waldie, "Los Angeles' Toilet-to-Tap Fear Factor," *Los Angeles Times,* December 1, 2002.

16. Orange County Water District, *A History of Orange County Water District, 2nd edition* (Tustin, CA: Acorn Group, 2014), 19.

17. Bob D. Newport, *Salt Water Intrusion in the United States, EPA 600/8-77-011* (Ada, OK: Robert S. Kerr Environmental Research Laboratory, Office of Research and Development, US Environmental Protection Agency, July 1977), 2–4.

18. Orange County Water District, *A History of Orange County Water District,* 10–14; Lassiter, *Sustainable Water: Challenges and Solutions from California,* 224.

19. Mike Wehner, author's interview, December 18, 2017.

20. Orange County Water District, *A History of Orange County Water District,* 36–38.

21. Mike Wehner, email to the author, August 28, 2018. As groundwater extraction grew, the salt intrusion was slowed by pumping yet more freshwater into the barrier.

22. Perry McCarty et al., "Advanced Treatment for Wastewater Reclamation at Water Factory 21," Stanford University, Department of Civil Engineering, Grant No. EPA-CS-806736-01-3 (August 1982), 2, summarized in Perry McCarty et al., *Project Summary: Advanced Treatment for Wastewater Reclamation at Water Factory 21, EPA 600/S2-84-031* (Cincinnati: US Environmental Protection Agency, Municipal Environmental Research Laboratory, February 1984), 2.

23. Orange County Water District, *A History of Orange County Water District,* 36.

24. Ibid., 50.

25. Michael R. Markus, author's interview, March 22, 2017.

26. Ibid.

27. Eleanor Torres, email to the author, December 27, 2017.

28. US Environmental Protection Agency, "EPA Provides $135 Million for Innovative Groundwater Replenishment Project Expansion in Orange County, California," press release, US EPA Press Office, August 1, 2018.

29. "WaterSense: How We Use Water," US Environmental Protection Agency, accessed April 30, 2018: https://www.epa.gov/watersense/how-we-use-water.

30. Gerald A Silver, author's interview, December 19, 2017; Forest Tennant, author's interview, February 10, 2018.

31. Marti Emerald, author's interview, December 22, 2017.

32. Michael R. Markus, author's interview, March 22, 2017.

33. Eleanor Torres, email to the author, August 31, 2018.

34. Mike Wehner, author's interview, December 18, 2017.

35. Mike Wehner, email to the author, August 28, 2018.

36. Ibid.

37. Eleanor Torres, email to the author, January 14, 2019.

38. Mike Wehner, author's interview, June 1, 2017.

TEN: NEW IDEAS NEEDED

1. National Vital Statistics Reports, Vol. 50, No. 6, "Life Expectancy at Birth, by Race and Sex, Selected Years 1929–98": Life expectancy differs by sex and race. From 1900 to 1950, life expectancy for white men increased by 43 percent; for white women, 47 percent; for black men, 79 percent; and black women, 85 percent. Because of the effects of racial discrimination on the health and safety of black Americans, and therefore on their longevity, the effect of cleaner drinking water may not be as clear as compared to white men and women. Still, there is little doubt that black Americans were also beneficiaries of cleaner water in that same half century.

2. David M. Cutler and Grant Miller, "The Role of Public Health Improvements in Health Advances: The Twentieth-Century United States," *Demography* 42, no. 1 (February 2005), 3.

3. Jeffrey Griffiths, author's interview, April 15, 2018.

4. Frost and Sullivan, *Global Outlook of the Water Industry, 2018* (San Antonio: Frost & Sullivan, 2018).

5. Seth M. Siegel, *Let There Be Water: Israel's Solution for a Water-Starved World* (New York: St. Martin's Press, 2015), 167–68.

6. For bottled water disposable bottles, see "Fact Sheet: Single-Use Plastics," Earth Day Network, accessed January 7, 2019: https://www.earthday.org/2018/03/29/fact-sheet -single-use-plastics/#_ftn4. For plastic containers more generally, the recycling rate is under 10 percent. See Roland Geyer et al., "Production, Use, and Fate of All Plastics Ever Made," *Science Advances* 3, no. 7 (July 2017).

7. Maura Allaire et al., "National Trends in Drinking Water Quality Violations," *PNAS* 115, no. 9 (February 2018): 2081.

8. Many cities, such as Milwaukee and Saint Paul, among others, already host "open door" events at their water utilities, allowing consumers to visit and learn about how their water is treated.

9. American Society of Civil Engineers, *2017 Infrastructure Report Card: Drinking Water* (Reston, VA: American Society of Civil Engineers, 2017), 1.

10. "Utility Rate Database," OpenEI, accessed January 3, 2018: https://openei.org/wiki/Utility_Rate_Database.

11. "Cable Internet Providers," BroadbandNOW, accessed January 3, 2018: https://broadbandnow.com/Cable-Providers.

12. "Directory of Representatives," US House of Representatives, accessed January 3, 2018: https://www.house.gov/representatives.

13. "How Many Counties Are There in the United States?," US Geological Survey, accessed January 3, 2019: https://www.usgs.gov/faqs/how-many-counties-are-there-united-states.

14. American Water Works Association, *2015 AWWA State of the Water Industry Report* (Denver: American Water Works Association, 2015), 11.

15. Joseph Kane and Adie Tomer, *Renewing the Water Workplace: Improving Water Infrastructure and Creating a Pipeline to Opportunity* (Washington, DC: Metropolitan Policy Program at Brookings, June 2018), 6; Elizabeth Douglass, "Towns Sell Their Public Water Systems—And Come to Regret It," *Washington Post,* July 8, 2017.

16. Felicia Marcus, author's interview, September 21, 2018.

17. Joseph Ayotte et al., "Estimating the High-Arsenic Domestic-Well Population in the Conterminous United States," *Environmental Science and Technology* 51 (2017): 12443: 54.

18. "Private Wells," US Environmental Protection Agency, accessed November 5, 2018: https://www.epa.gov/privatewells.

19. US Geological Survey (USGS), *Estimated Use of Water in the United States in 2015, Circular 1441* (Reston, VA: US Geological Survey, 2017), 22.

20. Leslie A. DeSimone, *Quality of Water from Domestic Wells in Principal Aquifers of the United States, 1991–2004, Scientific Investigations Report 2008–5227* (Reston, VA: US Geological Survey, 2009), 9, 17–57.

21. Lee Bergquist, "Study Shows Widespread Well Contamination in Southwestern Wisconsin," *Milwaukee Journal Sentinel,* January 2, 2019.

22. Margaret McCasland et al., *Nitrate: Health Effects in Drinking Water* (Ithaca, NY: Cornell University, Cooperative Extension, 2012).

23. Jay Fletcher and Weldon Freeman, *USDA Invests $256 Million in Water Infrastructure in Rural Communities,* press release no. 0115.18 (Washington, DC: US Department of Agriculture, May 23, 2018).

24. Ayotte et. al, "Estimating the High-Arsenic Domestic-Well Population in the Conterminous United States."

25. Troy Cook et al., "Hydraulically Fractured Horizontal Wells Account for Most New

Oil and Natural Gas Wells," *US Energy Information Administration, Today In Energy,* January 30, 2018.

26. Amy Mall, author's interview, November 2, 2018.

27. Jeff Kart, "EPA, Israeli Company Partner on 'Water from Air' Tech," *Forbes,* April 13, 2018.

28. Jim Elder, author's interview, April 16, 2018.

29. Henry Waxman, author's interview, January 30, 2018.

30. Although it is different in many ways, the independence of the National Academies of Sciences, Engineering, and Medicine is a model for how drinking water could be insulated from political pressure.

31. In what may be an important turning point, the EPA may be going ahead with the regulation of PFAS, even though it may have a large budgetary impact on the Pentagon. Julie Turkewitz, "'Stabbed in the Back': Polluted Water Pains Military Families," *New York Times,* February 23, 2019, A10.

32. US Environmental Protection Agency, Fiscal Year 2019 Justification of Appropriation Estimates for the Committee on Appropriations, EPA-190-R-18-001, 133.

33. Erik Olson, email to author, February 28, 2019.

34. As a few examples: The EPA set an MCL standard for arsenic at 50 ppb (1975), but lowered it to 10 ppb (2001). (Mark R. Powell, *Science at the EPA,* (Washington, DC: Resources for the Future, 1999), 196). The EPA set an MCL standard for lead at 50 ppb (1975), but lowered it to 15 ppb (1991) (*Science at the EPA,* 160–161). While PFOA is not regulated, the EPA issued a health advisory of 400 ppt (2009), but following interim steps of 200 and 100 ppt, ultimately lowered it to 70 ppt (2016) (US Environmental Protection Agency, *Provisional Health Advisories for Perfluorooctanoic Acid (PFOA) and Perfluorooctane Sulfonate (PFOS),* January 8, 2009; US Environmental Protection Agency, *Fact Sheet: PFOA & PFOS Drinking Water Health Advisories, EPA 800-F-16-003,* November 2016).

35. Gary Hemphill, Managing Director of Research, Beverage Marketing Corporation, email to the author, July 2, 2018

36. Robert Brutvan, "Taxes Will Account for Nearly One-Third of Chicago's Soda Prices," *Illinois Policy,* June 28, 2017.

37. "The USGS Water Science School: Water Questions and Answers," US Geological Survey, accessed January 3, 2019: https://water.usgs.gov/edu/qa-home-percapita.html.

38. *Safe Drinking Water Act Amendments of 1996,* 42 U.S.C. 300f-300j, as amended by P.L. 104–182. "Unregulated Contaminants," §1445 (42 U.S.C. 300j-4).

39. *Safe Drinking Water Act Amendments of 1996,* "Enforcement of Drinking Water Regulations," §1414 (42 U.S.C. 300g-3).

40. Food and Water Watch, *America's Secret Water Crisis: National Shut Off Survey Reveals Water Affordability Emergency Affecting Millions* (Washington, DC: Food and Water Watch, 2018).

41. US Environmental Protection Agency, *Drinking Water and Waste Water Utility Customer Assistance Programs* (Washington, DC: US Environmental Protection Agency, April 2016), 6.

Selected Bibliography

TO SEE THE COMPLETE BIBLIOGRAPHY,
PLEASE VISIT WWW.TROUBLEDWATER.US.

BOOKS

Adams, John H., and Patricia Adams. *A Force for Nature: The Story of the NRDC and the Fight to Save Our Planet.* San Francisco: Chronicle Books, 2010.

Brandt, Malcolm J., K. Michael Johnson, Andrew J. Elphinston, and Don D. Ratnayaka. *Twort's Water Supply,* 6th edition. Oxford, UK: Elsevier, 2009.

Carson, Rachel L. *Silent Spring.* New York: Houghton Mifflin Harcourt, 2002; originally published 1962.

Christian-Smith, Juliet, and Peter H. Gleick. *A Twenty-First Century U.S. Water Policy.* New York: Oxford University Press, 2012.

Clark, Anna. *The Poisoned City: Flint's Water and the American Urban Tragedy.* New York: Metropolitan Books/Henry Holt, 2018.

Drinan, Joanne E., and Nancy E. Whiting. *Water and Wastewater Treatment: A Guide for the Nonengineering Professional.* Boca Raton, FL: CRC Press, 2001.

Egan, Dan. *The Death and Life of the Great Lakes.* New York: W. W. Norton, 2017.

Fetter, Charles Willard. *Applied Hydrogeology.* 4th edition. Upper Saddle River, NJ: Prentice Hall, 2014.

Hanna-Attisha, Mona. *What the Eyes Don't See: A Story of Crisis, Resistance, and Hope in an American City.* New York: One World, 2018.

Hiltzik, Michael. *Colossus: Hoover Dam and the Making of the American Century.* New York: Free Press, 2010.

Johnson, Steven. *The Ghost Map: The Story of London's Most Terrifying Epidemic—And How It Changed Science, Cities, and the Modern World*. New York: Riverhead Books, 2007.

Koeppel, Gerard T. *Water for Gotham: A History*. Princeton: Princeton University Press, 2000.

McGuire, Michael J. *The Chlorine Revolution: Water Disinfection and the Fight to Save Lives*. Denver: American Water Works Association, 2013.

Melosi, Martin V. *Precious Commodity: Providing Water for America's Cities*. Pittsburgh: University of Pittsburgh Press, 2011.

Milazzo, Paul C. *Unlikely Environmentalists: Congress and Clean Water, 1945–1972*. Lawrence: University Press of Kansas, 2006.

Pontius, Frederick W. *Drinking Water Regulation and Health*. New York: John Wiley & Sons, 2003.

Powell, Mark R. *Science at the EPA: Information in the Regulatory Process*. Washington, DC: Resources for the Future, 1999.

Salzman, James. *Drinking Water: A History*. New York: Overlook Duckworth, 2012.

Siegel, Seth M. *Let There Be Water: Israel's Solution for a Water-Starved World*. New York: St. Martin's Press, 2015.

Solomon, Steven. *Water: The Epic Struggle for Wealth, Power, and Civilization*. New York: HarperCollins, 2010.

Speth, J. Gustave. *Angels by the River*. White River Junction, VT: Chelsea Green Publishing, 2014.

Tarr, Joel. *The Search for the Ultimate Sink: Urban Pollution in Historical Perspective*. Akron, OH: University of Akron Press, 1996.

Troesken, Werner. *The Great Lead Water Pipe Disaster*. Cambridge: MIT Press, 2006.

Wagner, Martin, and Scott Lambert. *Freshwater Microplastics: Emerging Environmental Contaminants?* Cham, Switzerland: Springer, 2018.

LAWS AND REGULATIONS

Comprehensive Environmental Response, Compensation, and Liabilities Act (Superfund Law). 42 U.S.C. §9601 et seq. (1980).

"Federal Regulation of Bottled Water," Food and Drug Administration, Department of Health and Human Services. *21 CFR Chapter I, Subchapter B, Part 165—Beverages*.

Federal Water Pollution Control Act (Clean Water Act). 33 U.S.C. §§1251–1387 (1972).

The Frank Lautenberg Chemical Safety for the 21st Century Act. 15 U.S.C. ch. 53, subch. I §§2601–2629, as amended by P.L. 114–182.

Microbead-Free Waters Act of 2015. 21 U.S.C. §331 (2015).

Registration, Evaluation, Authorization and Restriction of Chemicals (REACH). EC 1907/2006.

Resource Conservation and Recovery Act (RCRA). 42 U.S.C. ch. 82 §6901 et seq. (1976).

Safe Drinking Water Act (SDWA). 42 U.S.C. §300f–300j (1974).

Safe Drinking Water Act Amendments of 1986. 42 U.S.C. §300f–300j, as amended by P.L. 99–339.

Safe Drinking Water Act Amendments of 1996. 42 U.S.C. §300f–300j, as amended by P.L. 104–182.

Toxic Substances Control Act (TSCA). 15 U.S.C. ch. 53, subch. I §§2601–2629 (1976).

JOURNALS AND EXTENDED ARTICLES

Allaire, Maura, Haowei Wu, and Upmanu Lall. "National Trends in Drinking Water Quality Violations." *PNAS* 115, no. 9 (February 27, 2018): 2078–83.

Arnnok, Prapha, Randolph R. Singh, Rodjana Burakham, Alicia Pérez-Fuentetaja, and Diana S. Aga. "Select Uptake and Bioaccumulation of Antidepressants in Fish from Effluent-Impacted Niagara River." *Environmental Science & Technology* 51 (2017): 10652–62.

Arvai, Antonette, Gary Klecka, Saad Jasim, Henryk Melcer, and Michael T. Laitta. "Protecting Our Great Lakes: Assessing the Effectiveness of Wastewater Treatments for the Removal of Chemicals of Emerging Concern." *Water Quality Research Journal of Canada* 49, no. 1 (2014): 23–31.

Ayotte, Joseph D., Laura Medalie, Sharon L. Qi, Lorraine C. Backer, and Bernard T. Nolan. "Estimating the High-Arsenic Domestic-Well Population in the Conterminous United States." *Environmental Science and Technology* 51 (2017): 12443–54

Blazer, Vicki S., Luke R. Iwanowicz, Holly Henderson, Patricia M. Mazik, Jill A. Jenkins, David A. Alvarez, and John A. Young. "Reproductive Endocrine Disruption in Smallmouth Bass (Micropterus Dolomieu) in the Potomac River Basin: Spatial and Temporal Comparisons of Biological Effects." *Environmental Monitoring and Assessment* 184 (2012): 4309–34.

Bove, Frank, Youn Shim, and Perri Zeitz, "Drinking Water Contaminants and Adverse Pregnancy Outcomes: A Review." *Environmental Health Perspectives* 110, no. 1 (February 2002): 61–74.

Brandhuber, Philip, Sarah Clark, and Kevin Morley. "A Review of Perchlorate Occurrence in Public Drinking Water Systems." *Journal AWWA* 101, no. 11 (November 2009): 63–73.

Byers, Randolph K., and Elizabeth E. Lord. "Late Effects of Lead Poisoning on Mental Development." *Journal of Diseases of Children* 66, no. 5 (1943): 471–94

Diduch, Malwina, Zaneta Polkowska, and Jacek Namiesnik. "Chemical Quality of Bottled Waters: A Review." *Journal of Food Science* 76, no. 9 (November 9, 2011): R178–R196.

Edwards, Marc. "Fetal Death and Reduced Birth Rates Associated with Exposure to Lead-Contaminated Drinking Water." *Environmental Science & Technology* 48 (2014): 739–46.

Grandjean, Philippe, and Richard Clapp. "Perfluorinated Alkyl Substances: Emerging Insights into Health Risks," *New Solutions* 25, no. 2 (June 17, 2015): 147–63.

Guart, Albert, Martin Wagner, Alejandro Mezquida, Silvia Lacorte, Jörg Oehlmann, and Antonio Borrell. "Migration of Plasticisers from Tritan and Polycarbonate Bottles and Toxicological Evaluation." *Food Chemistry* 141 (2013): 373–80.

Iwanowicz, L., V. S. Blazer, A. E. Pinkney, C. P. Guy, A. M. Major, K. Munney, S. Mierzykowski, S. Lingenfelser, A. Secord, K. Patnode, T. J. Kubiak, C. Stern, C. M. Hahn, D. D. Iwanowicz, H. L. Walsh, and A. Sperry. "Evidence of Estrogenic Endocrine Disruption in Smallmouth and Largemouth Bass Inhabiting Northeast U.S. National Wildlife Refuge Waters: A Reconnaissance Study." *Ecotoxicology and Environmental Safety* 124 (2016): 50–59.

Jobling, Susan, S. Coey, J. G. Whitmore, D. E. Kime, K. J. W. Van Look, B. G. McAllister, N. Beresford, A. C. Henshaw, G. Brighty, C. R. Tyler, and J. P. Sumpter. "Wild Intersex Roach (*Rutilus rutilus*) Have Reduced Fertility." *Biology of Reproduction* 67, no. 2 (2002): 515–24.

Jones, Steven M., Zaid K. Chowdhury, and Michael J. Watts. "A Taxonomy of *Chemicals of Emerging Concern* Based on Observed Fate at Water Resource Recovery Facilities." *Chemosphere* 170 (2017): 153–60.

Kolodziej, Edward P., and David L. Sedlak. "Rangeland Grazing as a Source of Steroid Hormones to Surface Waters." *Environmental Science & Technology* 41, no. 10 (April 14, 2007): 3514–20.

Kosuth, Mary, Sherri A. Mason, and Elizabeth V. Wattenberg. "Anthropogenic Contamination of Tap Water, Beer, and Sea Salt." *PLoS ONE* 13, no. 4 (April 2018): e0194970.

Leung, Angela M., Elizabeth N. Pearce, and Lewis E. Braverman. "Perchlorate, Iodine and the Thyroid." *Best Practice & Research: Clinical Endocrinology & Metabolism* 24, no. 1 (2010): 133–41.

McGuire, Michael J. "Eight Revolutions in the History of US Drinking Water Disinfection." *Journal AWWA* 98, no. 3 (March 2006): 123–49.

Needleman, Herbert L., and David Bellinger; "The Health Effect of Low-Level Exposure to Lead." *Annual Review of Public Health* 12 (1991): 123.

Needleman, Herbert L., Christine McFarland, Roberta B. Ness, Stephen E. Fienberg, and Michael J. Tobin. "Bone Lead Levels in Adjudicated Delinquents." *Neurotoxicology & Teratology* 24, no. 6 (November–December 2002): 711–17.

Okun, Daniel A. "From Cholera to Cancer to Cryptosporidiosis." *Journal of Environmental Engineering* 122, no. 6 (June 1996): 453–58.

Olson, Erik D. "The Quiet Shift of Power: Office of Management and Budget Supervision of Environmental Protection Agency Rulemaking under Executive Order 12,291." *Virginia Journal of Natural Resources Law* 4, no. 1 (1984).

Pearce, Elizabeth N., John H. Lazarus, Rodrigo Moreno-Reyes, and Michael B. Zimmermann. "Consequences of Iodine Deficiency and Excess in Pregnant Women: An Overview of Current Knowns and Unknowns." *The American Journal of Clinical Nutrition* 104, no. 3 (September 2016): 919–23.

Phillips, P. J., C. Schubert, D. Argue, I. Fisher, E. T. Furlong, W. Foreman, J. Gray, and A. Chalmers. "Concentrations of Hormones, Pharmaceuticals, and Other Micropollutants in Groundwater Affected by Septic Systems in New England and New York." *Science of the Total Environment* 512–13 (2015): 43–54.

Rochester, Johanna R. "Bisphenol A and Human Health: A Review of the Literature." *Reproductive Toxicology* 42 (December 2013): 132–55.

Sass, Jennifer. "U.S. Department of Defense and White House Working Together to Avoid Liability for Perchlorate Pollution." *International Journal of Occupational and Environmental Health* (2004): 330–34.

Schymanski, Darena, Christophe Goldbeck, Hans-Ulrich Humpf, and Peter Fürst. "Analysis of Microplastics in Water by Micro-Raman Spectroscopy: Release of Plastic Particles from Different Packaging into Mineral Water." *Water Research* 129 (November 2017): 154–62.

Simons, Joseph. "The Seven Ages of Fluorine Chemistry." *Journal of Fluorine Chemistry* 32 (1986): 7–24.

Stanbury, John, and James Wyngaarden. "Effect of Perchlorate on the Human Thyroid Gland." *Metabolism* 1, no. 6 (November 1952): 533–39.

Steinmaus, Craig, Michelle Pearl, Martin Kharrazi, Benjamin C. Blout, Mark D. Miller, Elizabeth N. Pearce, Liza Valentin-Blasini, Gerald DeLorenze, Andrew N. Hoofnagle, and Jane Liaw. "Thyroid Hormones and Moderate Exposure to Perchlorate During Pregnancy in Women in Southern California." *Environmental Health Perspectives* 124, no. 6 (2016): 861–67.

Symons, George E. "Water Treatment Through the Ages." *Journal AWWA* 98, no. 3 (March 2006): 87–98.

Symons, James. "The Early History of Disinfection By-Products: A Personal Chronicle—Part 1." *Environmental Engineer* 37, no. 1 (January 2001): 21–25.

Verlicchi, Paola, A. Galletti, M. Petrovic, and D. Barceló. "Hospital Effluents as a Source of Emerging Pollutants: An Overview of Micropollutants and Sustainable Treatment Options." *Journal of Hydrology* 389 (2010): 416–28.

Wagner, Martin. Michael P. Schlüsener, Thomas A. Ternes, and Jörg Oehlmann. "Identification of Putative Steroid Receptor Antagonists in Bottled Water: Combining Bioassays and High-Resolution Mass Spectrometry." *PLoS ONE* 8, no. 8 (August 2013).

Wasserstrom, Lauren W., Stephanie A. Miller, Simoni Triantafyllidou, Michael DeSantis, and Michael Schock. "Scale Formation Under Blended Phosphate Treatment for a Utility with Lead Pipes." *Journal AWWA* 109, no. 11 (November 2017): E464–E478.

Zimmer, J. L., R. M. Slawson, and P. M. Huck. "Inactivation and Potential Repair of *Cryptosporidium Parvum* Following Low-and Medium-Pressure Ultraviolet Irradiation." *Water Research* 37, no. 14 (August 2003): 3517–23.

Zoeller, R. Thomas, T. R. Brown, L. L. Doan, A. C. Gore, N. E. Skakkebaek, A. M. Soto, T. J. Woodruff, and F. S. Vom Saal. "Endocrine-Disrupting Chemicals and Public Health Protection: A Statement of Principles from the Endocrine Society." *Endocrinology* 153, no. 9 (2012): 4097–4110.

REPORTS

Agency for Toxic Substances and Disease Registry. *Public Health Statement: Vinyl Chloride, CAS#: 75-01-4.* Atlanta: US Department of Health and Human Services, July 2006.

Agency for Toxic Substances and Disease Registry. *Public Health Statement on Perchlorates.* Atlanta: US Department of Health and Human Services, September 2008.

Agency for Toxic Substances Disease Registry. *Toxicological Profile for Perfluoroalkyls, Draft for Public Comment.* Atlanta: US Department of Health and Human Services, June 2018.

American Society of Civil Engineers. *2017 Infrastructure Report Card: A Comprehensive Assessment of America's Infrastructure.* Reston, VA: American Society of Civil Engineers, 2017.

American Water Works Association. *Dawn of the Replacement Era: Reinvesting in Drinking Water Infrastructure.* Denver: American Water Works Association, May 2001.

American Water Works Association. *Buried No Longer: Confronting America's Water Infrastructure Challenge.* Denver: American Water Works Association, February 27, 2012.

American Water Works Association. *2015 AWWA State of the Water Industry Report.* Denver: American Water Works Association, 2015.

American Water Works Association. *The State of Water Loss Control in Drinking Water Utilities,* White Paper. Denver: American Water Works Association, 2016.

Cutler, David, and Grant Miller. *The Role of Public Health Improvements in Health Advances: The 20th Century United States.* Harvard University, February 2004.

DeSimone, Leslie A. *Quality of Water from Domestic Wells in Principal Aquifers of the United States, 1991–2004, Scientific Investigations Report 2008–5227.* Reston, VA: US Geological Survey, 2009.

Drinking Water Research Foundation. *Bottled Water and Tap Water: Just the Facts—A Comparison of Regulatory Requirements for Quality and Monitoring of Drinking Water in the United States.* Alexandria, VA: Drinking Water Research Foundation, March 2014.

Environmental Working Group. *Pesticides in Baby Food.* Washington, DC: Environmental Working Group, July 1, 1995.

Fedinick, Kristi Pullen, Mae Wu, Mekela Panditharatne, and Erik D. Olson. *Threats on Tap:*

Widespread Violations Highlight Need for Investment in Water Infrastructure and Protections. Washington, DC: Natural Resources Defense Council, May 2017.

Johnson, Kenneth. *Demographic Trends in Rural and Small Town America*. Durham: University of New Hampshire, Carsey Institute, 2006.

Lai, Larry. *Adopting County Policies Which Limit Public Water System Sprawl and Promote Small System Consolidation*. Los Angeles: University of California, Los Angeles, Luskin School of Public Affairs, May 2017.

Levin, Ronnie. *Reducing Lead in Drinking Water: A Benefit Analysis. EPA 230-09-86-019*. Washington, DC: US Environmental Protection Agency, December 1986 (revised, Spring 1987).

McCarty, Perry L., Martin Reinhard, Naomi L. Goodman, James W. Graydon, Gary D. Hopkins, Kristien E. Mortelmans, and David G. Argo. *Project Summary: Advanced Treatment for Wastewater Reclamation at Water Factory 21, EPA 600/S2-84-031*. Cincinnati: US Environmental Protection Agency, Municipal Environmental Research Laboratory, February 1984.

Mushak, Paul, Matthew McKinzie, and Erik Olson. *Arsenic and Old Laws: A Scientific and Public Health Analysis of Arsenic Occurrence in Drinking Water, Its Health Effects, and EPA's Outdated Arsenic Tap Water Standard*. Washington, DC: Natural Resources Defense Council, February 2000.

National Academy of Sciences. *Health Implications of Perchlorate Ingestion*. Washington, DC: National Academies Press, 2005.

National Center for Health Statistics. *Health, United States, 2016: With Chartbook on Long-term Trends in Health*. Hyattsville, MD: US Department of Health and Human Services, 2017.

National Wildlife Federation. *Danger on Tap: The Government's Failure to Enforce the Federal Safe Drinking Water Act, FY 1988 Update*. Washington, DC: National Wildlife Federation, Environmental Quality Division, 1989.

Natural Resources Defense Council. *Victorian Water Treatment Enters the 21st Century: Public Health Threats from Water Utilities' Ancient Treatment and Distribution Systems*. Washington, DC: Natural Resources Defense Council, March 1994.

Office of Water Services (Ofwat). *The Development of the Water Industry in England and Wales*. Birmingham, UK: Ofwat, 2006.

Olson, Erik D. *Think Before You Drink: The Failure of the Nation's Drinking Water System to Protect Public Health*. Washington, DC: Natural Resources Defense Council, September 1993.

Olson, Erik D. *Bottled Water: Pure Drink or Pure Hype?* Washington DC: Natural Resources Defense Council, February 1999, Updated Commentary, September 2, 2010.

Olson, Erik, and Kristi Pullen Fedinick. *What's in Your Water? Flint and Beyond: Analysis of EPA Data Reveals Widespread Lead Crisis Potentially Affecting Millions of Americans*. Washington, DC: Natural Resources Defense Council, 2016.

Orange County Water District. *A History of Orange County Water District,* 2nd edition. Tustin, CA: Acorn Group, 2014.

Pharmaceutical Input and Elimination from Local Sources (PILLS). *Pharmaceutical Residues in the Aquatic System—A Challenge for the Future.* Gelsenkirchen, Germany: PILLS, September 2012.

Tiemann, Mary. *Safe Drinking Water Act (SDWA): A Summary of the Act and Its Major Requirements.* Washington, DC: Congressional Research Service, Library of Congress, March 2017.

US Centers for Disease Control and Prevention. *Antibiotic Use in the United States, 2017: Progress and Opportunities.* Atlanta: US Department of Health and Human Services, 2017.

US Environmental Protection Agency, Office of Water. *25 Years of the Safe Drinking Water Act: History and Trends.* Washington, DC: US Environmental Protection Agency, December 1999.

US Environmental Protection Agency. *Variances and Exemptions: A Quick Reference Guide, EPA 816-F-04-005.* Washington, DC: US Environmental Protection Agency, Office of Water, September 2004.

US Environmental Protection Agency. *Lead and Copper Rule Monitoring and Reporting Guidance for Public Water Systems, EPA 816-R-10-004.* Washington, DC: US Environmental Protection Agency, revised March 2010.

US Environmental Protection Agency. *Drinking Water: EPA Needs to Take Additional Steps to Ensure Small Community Water Systems Designated as Serious Violators Achieve Compliance, Report No. 16-P-0108.* Washington, DC: US Environmental Protection Agency, March 22, 2016.

US Environmental Protection Agency. *Lead and Copper Rule Revisions White Paper.* Washington, DC: US Environmental Protection Agency, Office of Water, October 2016.

US Environmental Protection Agency. *Drinking Water Infrastructure Needs Survey and Assessment, Sixth Report to Congress, EPA 816-K-17-002.* Washington, DC: US Environmental Protection Agency, March 2018.

US Geological Survey. *Estimated Use of Water in the United States in 2015, Circular 1441.* Reston, VA: US Geological Survey, 2017.

W. K. Kellogg Foundation, prepared by the Horsley Witten Group, Inc. *Managing Lead in Drinking Water at Schools and Early Childhood Education Facilities.* Battle Creek, MI: W. K. Kellogg Foundation, February 2016.

Index